Killing Leuk

ISBN: 1542726166
ISBN 13: 9781542726160

Library of Congress Control Number: 2017901197
CreateSpace Independent Publishing Platform
North Charleston, South Carolina

Contents

One

It was an unusually sunny day for February in Alaska. My three children and I were standing in the backyard, and we were filled with happiness. Our joy radiated through the picture I took that day on February 12, 1997. The kids were wearing big wax lips their grandma Michele had sent them from Colorado. They were being goofy, and I was proud to be their mom. Suddenly, a dark cloud formed. It wasn't visible, but I could feel it. I heard God say to me, "Will you still love me when your life dramatically changes?" They weren't audible words, but they were clearly words that penetrated my thought process. Suddenly, I knew that something bad was going to happen.

I tried to shake off that uneasy feeling. What possibly could go wrong with our perfect little family? Patrick and I had met during my senior year of high school. He had graduated from a Colorado high school the year before and had come to Alaska for the fishing trip that never ended. I moved up in 1983, when I was going into my junior year of high school. My dad had pastored a church for years in Indiana, and he had decided it was time to go somewhere else. He looked at a church in Texas, but I suggested he try Alaska. "Alaska?" he'd said. "I don't even like the cold!" I had extended family here, and it seemed so adventurous and impressive to say I was moving to Alaska! Sure enough, Dad applied to a church in Wasilla and was offered the position. We left the only state I knew and soon were driving thousands of miles north.

Thankfully, my granny, aunt, uncle, brother, and cousins all agreed to come too. What a sight to behold as the Oathouts traveled the Alcan in a large caravan. One rollover, multiple flat tires, and several muddy vehicles later, we arrived in Wasilla, Alaska. There was just one stoplight in the small town. We lived in our travel trailer parked outside the church for a while until we were offered a house-sitting position in Big Lake. I remember walking to the school bus one morning in high heels when there was about two feet of snow on the ground. I wanted to be "cool" as I went to this new school where I knew no one. I made several friends but was never asked out on a date by anyone! I wanted so badly to be loved by someone, as all the other girls seemed to be.

It wasn't till almost the end of my senior year that I met my future husband, Patrick. As soon as I saw him, I was struck with a feeling he would change my life. He walked into the room with his wavy red hair, wearing a jean jacket, looking like a sexy "bad boy." I felt a wave of attraction that I had never felt before. We dated off and on for a few months. He made it clear that we belonged together, but I wasn't ready to admit it. On June 27, 1985, another revelation hit me. I realized he was the one I wanted to spend the rest of my life with. He treated me with love and respect, and no matter how much I pushed him away, he was patiently waiting for me to admit I had fallen in love with him. I was only eighteen years old, but I knew I would never find a man who loved me as much as he did.

I did what everyone expected of me, though; I enrolled at the University of Alaska in Anchorage to study nursing. Back in 1979, Granny had planted the idea in my head that I should be a nurse. I had had some crazy medical things happen to me in my short lifetime. The first was when I was diagnosed with encephalitis at the age of six. Encephalitis is an inflammation of the brain and is usually spread by insects or animals. I remember Granny becoming hysterical at the hospital. I didn't understand why she was so upset. Later I learned that her youngest son, my uncle Dana, had died when he was four years old from encephalitis. Granny thought I was going to die too.

When I was twelve, my left jaw swelled up so badly that I looked like a chipmunk. I could barely open my mouth, and all my food had to be pureed. Try eating pureed steak; it's disgusting. My parents took me to several doctors, and no one knew what was wrong with me. They suspected bone cancer. I was referred to Mayo Clinic in Rochester, Minnesota. Almost immediately, they diagnosed me with osteomyelitis of the left mandible. Osteomyelitis is an inflammation of bone. It's a very rare occurrence to have this disease, but even rarer to have it in the jaw bone. I am nothing, if not unique. They surgically scraped my mandible of all the infection. Granny vowed to do the only thing I had ever asked her to do-stop smoking. She was so thankful that I was going to live, that she immediately stopped. I stayed in the hospital for almost a month. I was given large doses of cortisone, which caused my pancreas to "malfunction," and they temporarily put me on insulin. Afterward they just told me to watch my blood sugars. During my senior year, after a routine urinalysis, it became obvious that "watching my blood sugars" was not enough, and I went on insulin. After all this, Granny was convinced that I needed to be a nurse.

Like a dutiful granddaughter and daughter, I enrolled in college as directed. Unfortunately, besides not having a mind for chemistry, I was too much in love with Patrick to do much schoolwork. I dropped out after a semester and worked full time as an assistant manager of a popular clothing store. I was good at my job and loved the social aspect of it. Patrick and I drew closer and closer, and he proposed to me over grilled cheese and tomato soup on his lunch hour. It was an impromptu proposal, and there was no ring yet. I didn't care; I was on cloud nine! My parents were cautious, but they really didn't object. They liked Patrick because he showed them respect and treated me well. He faithfully went to church with me each week, and that made my parents very happy.

We had a beautiful wedding, six months later, at the Christian church my dad pastored. Mom made my wedding cake and bridesmaid dresses, and our friend Anita made my wedding dress. Everything was simply perfect.

After our marriage, we rented a house from Gary King, the father of one of Patrick's oldest friends, Tony. Patrick was working at Nye Ford, spraying rust-proofing materials on new vehicles, and I was working at a local clothing store. We didn't have a lot of money, but we were happy. Life was good, and we wanted to start a family right away. Within three months of marriage, I was pregnant. We were ecstatic! All our dreams were coming true. I was nineteen, and Patrick was twenty. People thought we were too young to start a family, but we knew what we were doing. We were young, happy, and in love.

Killing Leuk

Four days before our first anniversary, we welcomed our first-born son, Logan Joseph Marre, into the world at 7:44 a.m. on June 24, 1987. He was beautiful and perfect, and we were totally in love with him. Unfortunately, he was jaundiced and had to go back into the hospital for a few extra days. It was difficult to leave him at night. I wanted to be with him all the time. We were thankful when we got to bring him home and be a family. We doted on him and spent hours just admiring him. We had to fight off everyone in our family just to hold our son. He was a good-natured baby, and nothing seemed to faze him.

When Logan was two, we moved to Anchorage. Patrick was completing his prerequisites for occupational therapy at the University of Alaska and I was working full time at Sears. When he couldn't take care of Logan, my aunt Angie did. Life was good, and we didn't even think about having another child. One day I had some tests run because I wasn't feeling well. Were we ever surprised to find out I was pregnant! We simply had no idea. We were both shocked. I became very excited and drove right to my aunt's house to tell Logan. He was two and didn't really understand, but I wanted him to be the first to know. We elected not to find out the sex of this new baby. I think that was harder on my mom and me than on Patrick.

When our second son was born, I just laughed when I was told we had another boy. We decided to name him Casey. Whereas Logan was a sweet and calm boy, Casey was a wild and very active child. Their personalities were so different; there was never a dull moment in our household. Logan just loved Casey and took the role of big brother seriously. Whenever Casey would cry, I would put him in front of Logan, and Logan would play peek-a-boo with him and make him laugh. I decided not to go back to work after

Casey was born, so Patrick had to drop out of school and work full time. I felt bad about that, but there was no way we were going to have someone else raise our children.

It wasn't long before I was itching to have another baby. Two children were so much fun that I just knew I had to have another one. I don't remember ever telling Patrick about my deep desire to have another child because I didn't want him to obsess about it like I was. We had decided that two were plenty, and he got a vasectomy after Casey's birth. It was no longer possible to become pregnant—that is, until I prayed that God would *make* it possible. Sure enough, I became pregnant against all odds. I was simply having the time of my life. This time we found out ahead of time we were having a little girl. After two boys, I needed a girl!

After Meghan was born, Logan spoiled her rotten and protected her from eighteen-month-old Casey, who wanted to bang on her head with his hands like the *Flintstones* character, *Bam Bam.* Meghan was a sweet, beautiful little girl who had a touch of red hair like her daddy. Life seemed to be complete, and I had everything I wanted: a husband and three beautiful and healthy children.

As our children grew up, Casey followed Logan everywhere. When Logan wanted to hang out with friends, Casey was there. Sometimes Logan got irritated that he didn't get to spend much time without his brother, but he really did love the attention. They were as close as two brothers could be. Casey would crawl into bed with Logan each night.

We had bought a house in Wasilla when I was seven months pregnant with Meghan. We bought it at the tail end of the market this was happening. We met Logan's future doctor, Dr. Haydar Frangoul. Dr. Frangoul spoke with a heavy accent, but we immediately liked him and were reassured by his demeanor and willingness to explain the process.

Logan was admitted to the hospital, and tests were run. The diagnosis was confirmed: he had acute lymphocytic leukemia, also known as ALL or acute lymphoblastic leukemia. ALL is a cancer of the bone marrow, and Logan's bone marrow was making defective cells. I remember the nurses bringing a Charlie Brown movie into Logan's room, and the title was something like "What Does It Mean to Have Cancer?" I remember it was a few days before he would even watch it. He was angry. He said, "This sucks!" I had to chuckle, but being the mom I was, I still had to tell him that wasn't a nice word. Within a short time, a port was inserted into his chest so chemotherapy could be administered.

Little did I know that seventeen years later, I would also be told I had leukemia. My experience with Logan helped prepare me for my own battle.

Three

WHAT IS ALL?

We were told that ALL was the most common type of leukemia in children and the most curable. Logan seemed to be at a lower risk than many, and we were thrilled to think that he could beat this monster.

The standard treatment for ALL is a protocol that is divided into four phases. Each phase consists of heavy-duty chemotherapy tailored to fit the type of leukemia Logan had. The first phase is called *induction* and lasts about four weeks. The purpose of induction is to achieve remission, which is the absence of blast cells in the blood and bone marrow. After induction, there is *consolidation*, which is about twelve weeks long. Consolidation—it almost sounds easy, right? What it does is prepare the body for the difficult third phase, called *delayed intensification*. This is the stage when more intensive chemotherapy is given to the patient. I thought of it as a brutal wake-up after a bit of needed rest. It's an important phase, though, because those little devil cells must be destroyed. After successfully completing delayed intensification, the patient moves on to the *maintenance* phase. Girls usually spend two years on maintenance, and boys about three years.

We were informed that leukemia is a cancer of the bone marrow. The bone marrow makes three kinds of cells:

1. Red blood cells (RBC), which pick up oxygen and carry it to the tissues
2. Platelets, which are what helps stop bleeding when there is a cut
3. White blood cells (WBC), which are the infection-fighting cells

It's important to know what the WBC count is of a cancer patient so determination can be made about the advisability of being in risky situations such as crowds. If the white blood count is too low, patients are more susceptible to contracting illnesses such as a common cold or pneumonia. There are three main types of white blood cells:

*   Neutrophils (ANC), which eat bacteria
*   Lymphocytes, which make substances to fight bacteria
*   Monocytes, which destroy foreign materials

A blast cell is a short name for *lymphoblast*, the immature white blood cells. There are normal blasts and leukemic blasts. Blasts usually compose less than 5 percent of the cells made by the bone marrow and grow to form mature white blood cells. Leukemic blasts are abnormal because they don't mature and don't function like normal white blood cells.

We quickly learned the names of the chemotherapy drugs as well as how to administer various medications, what to look out for as far as signs of infections, and when to return to the hospital. We were told we always had to be within a few miles of the hospital during recovery after intensive chemotherapy. There was no telling when Logan's counts would drop, and if he spiked a fever, it would be an automatic admit to the hospital. We took the doctor's orders seriously and followed every precaution given. At times Logan was extremely sick. He was extremely fatigued and often nauseous. It was difficult to watch our active boy lose interest in normal daily activities. He had good days, though, when we would take many laps around the hospital corridors. Each day he soaked in the bathtub. The child loved baths! The housekeeping staff seemed a bit irritated with us because they had to clean the tub before he used it each day. We didn't care; he enjoyed his baths. He never seemed to feel too sick to play video games. He was no longer limited by his parents as to how much time he could spend gaming. We were much more lenient after he got sick.

We had to find a place to live while Logan was being treated. We were referred to Ronald McDonald House across the street from Children's Hospital. However, there were no openings at that time. We had to juggle housing arrangements until a room opened. It seemed unbelievable that so many children were so critically ill that there were not enough rooms for all the families. We quickly learned that many children had cancer, and some were even born with it! It was simply unfathomable that this could happen to us or to anyone else's child. Even today, twenty years past Logan's diagnosis date, I am still amazed at the number of children who have cancer.

Five

Our New Normal

We adjusted to hospital life the best we could. When we first arrived, they put us in a private room. After a few days, though, when things were sinking in, they moved us to a shared room. I don't remember the name of the boy who we shared with, but he was nice. His mother was older than I was and rather abrupt and a little bit rude. My husband used the restroom in the room, and she yelled that it was only for patients. I was still in shock and didn't realize that the phone was a shared line. I went to make a call, and she angrily told me she was on the phone and I had to wait my turn. I ran outside sobbing. When Patrick found me, I was crying about how I missed my kids, my dogs, my cats, and even our pet chicken! I was a sight to behold, for sure. I had hit my breaking point.

When Logan was released from the hospital, we had to go to the clinic almost every day for treatment or labs. One day, Logan was hoping his ANC (absolute neutrophil count) would be high enough so he could go to the mall without having to worry about fighting off germs. Unfortunately, it hadn't reached the minimum one thousand mark, so he couldn't go. On the return to Ronald McDonald House, he was kicking the gravel with his feet. I heard him mutter, "I'm just like a pit bull. You can't take me around people."

Despite the ups and downs and the scares we had, Logan did do well and went into remission in March. We got to come home for a bit on March 24. Things were going great. We had to go to Anchorage to see our wonderful pediatrician, Dr. Keller, for weekly chemo. We dreaded those Mondays. One time we had to pull over after driving on Trunk, which was a very curvy road. Logan was nauseous from his medication, and I got carsick driving. We both threw up alongside the road. I joked that my sympathy for how he felt made me sick too. Seventeen years later, I personally could understand how chemotherapy made a person nauseous.

We didn't like those Monday trips, but we enjoyed being together, and our bond grew stronger each week. I was always in awe of my boy. He was so brave! The boy who'd had to be held down for stitches became the bravest boy I have ever met in my life. He was simply amazing. Life was semi normal and good.

The year Logan was diagnosed, we had made the decision to homeschool our children. I was thrilled to be with them all the time and worked hard to maintain their schooling as best as I could. Logan was gifted in all subjects, but he particularly liked science.

Logan used to impress his doctors with questions about various things he had learned about his cells. They quickly realized they could not treat him like a child. They learned to talk with him about his illness without trying to sugarcoat it. I remember one new doctor who treated him like the child he was. Logan spouted off some intelligent comment, and the doctor said, "Okay, Logan, I see that you aren't really at a child's level, so I will make sure I don't treat you like a child." Logan was pretty impressed with himself.

Logan's tenth birthday was June 24. We had to be in Seattle for his actual birthday, so we had a party at Matanuska River Park before we left. His aunt and uncle gave him an awesome black mountain bike, and he rode it all around the park. Many friends and family members came to celebrate with him, and he was showered with love and presents.

One day, while riding bikes through our neighborhood, Logan said, "Mom, what percentage do I have to live?" I told him it didn't matter because he was going to beat leukemia no matter what. He insisted I tell him the truth. I told him that statistics showed that ALL had an 80 percent survival rate. He perked up and exclaimed, "Those are good odds" as he rode off happily ahead of me. Years later, my college statistics professor told our class how statistics lie and can be manipulated any which way. He was right.

Since we were in Seattle for Logan's actual birthday, we celebrated with a dinner at Ronald McDonald House with our friend Jeff, and then we took Logan to a drive-in theater in Auburn. Logan's favorite activity was watching movies. He loved to quote movie lines with Casey and Meghan. His favorite actors were Jim Carrey and Jackie Chan, and we would watch their movies over and over.

Six

STILL UNITED

On July 8, 1997, Logan made the decision to have his head shaved. For several days, his short brown hair had been falling out, and he was fed up with it. His friend Taylor, who also had ALL, came to our room at Ronald McDonald House with his dad, Marc. Marc shaved Logan's head. I remember being a wreck inside, wondering how he would accept this newest change in his life. Thankfully, our good-natured and brave son proudly displayed his bald head. Casey elected to shave his head as well. He was only six, and I was so amazed at his willingness to be comrades with his brother. What an act of love.

It was around this time when they had "Jay Buhner night" at the Mariners' game. Those who showed up with shaved heads got into the baseball game for free. Buhner was bald and kids were willing to shave their heads so they could be like their baseball hero. Before we went to a game, we went to a grocery store. Someone asked Logan and Taylor if they had shaved their heads for Buhner night. Logan elected to simply answer yes, while Taylor went into detail about their ALL diagnosis. Logan just wanted to be a normal boy who shaved his head to commemorate one of his favorite athletes.

We spent time participating in as many fun events as we could as a family. We wanted to show all three of the kids that despite Logan's diagnosis, we were still a family, and we cared about *each* of them.

Things were good until it was time for Logan to get his next round of chemo. He had a port in his chest, and we had to put Emla cream on it to numb it before accessing it for blood draws and chemotherapy. On July 21, I put the cream on too low, and it was very painful for Logan. He cried, I cried, and Meghan cried. I felt like the worst mother in the world. I had failed our boy. It was one of the hardest days he'd had up to that point.

The doctors allowed us to take Logan home to Alaska for a while. We settled back in as a family and again tried to normalize everything as much as possible. It was so important to both Patrick and me to make sure each child knew he or she was loved and valued by us.

We chose to let my mom take Logan down to Seattle for the first three weeks of his next round of chemo so I could stay with Casey and Meghan. I was hosting a Bible study while home, and when it came time for prayer requests, Logan asked for prayers for me to be okay while he was with his grandma at the hospital. Logan always put everyone else first.

During this time, we were spiritually attacked by the devil. Dad had flat tires, Mom's transmission went out, our car had a blown engine, and Logan was having more side effects from chemo, including tremors, vomiting, and a rash. Our beloved dog, Badger, was dying, and Logan didn't get to say good-bye to him. I made a note in my journal that when the devil strikes, he strikes hard, but God is stronger. Even after everything our family has gone through, I still believe that.

Logan ended up in the ICU when my mom took him down for that intensive chemo. My plans of staying in Alaska longer with Casey and Meghan came to a halt as I changed my ticket and got there as soon as I could. I was so torn between my children. All three of them needed me, but I had to be with Logan because he was so sick. He was tested for so many things and at one point was deprived of food for a few days. I remember our friends Waleen and Larry and Ginny and Ernie coming to see him and trying to distract him from his growling tummy.

Seven

There were months of ups and downs as Logan battled ALL with chemotherapy. Watching my child vomit and suffer was too much to bear. We got close to many families at Ronald McDonald House, and we were devastated whenever we learned of a child's death. I loved the camaraderie we all shared, but it was also painful. When a child died, not only did we grieve for the child and his or her parents, but we feared the same thing would happen to us. Would we lose our firstborn son? Surely not! He was way too strong to be beaten by leukemia.

We met several families from Anchorage while at Ronald McDonald House and Children's Hospital: Lake, Breanna, Ariel, Jordan, and Christopher. Lake, Ariel, and Christopher also had ALL, and Jordan and Breanna had rhabdomyosarcoma, which is a cancer of soft tissue. It usually begins in muscles that are attached to bones. We also met Chase from Soldotna, who had ALL. There were many others, but I have lost track of them over the years. We Alaskans stuck together and cheered each other on. Lake, Ariel, and Chase made it, and are doing fine to this day. Christopher, Breanna, and Jordan lost their valiant fights against cancer. I found out that a few years later Breanna's parents lost another child to the same cancer.

Every time another child died, I grieved the loss. I longed for a time when I was not affected by the death of a child. Losing a child is completely unnatural, and it is so wrong.

I remember one evening in Seattle when Logan started running a fever. It was just the two of us together at that time, and I had to take him to the hospital. He was very upset and wrote Patrick a note that said, "Dad, come quick! I have a fever and need to go to the hospital." I wanted to cry and laugh at the same time. I'm not sure how he thought his dad would read that note, because in those days we didn't have a cell phone we could use to text.

On October 27, 1997, Patrick wrote this letter to Logan:

Dear Logan,

Hey buddy, how are you doing? I was just thinking about you and thought, "I should write Logan a letter." I got to talk to you today, and that always makes me feel better. I can't wait until we are together again.

I wanted to tell you how proud of you I am, Logan. You have been faced with an incredible amount of challenge, more than I can handle, and you just keep kicking butt. It feels good to know that you are so strong and have the attitude to defeat this thing, and I know you will.

Logan, all your life you will be up against new and difficult challenges. Apply the same courage and strength you have shown this past year, and there won't be anything in this world that you can't do. (Plus, the girls will all fall in love with you!)

Write me a letter, and I will read it. There are so many things that I want to talk to you about, but my handwriting is not the best. So, if you write me back a short letter like this, then I will write back, and pretty soon we will have said a lot.

I love you son, and I am proud to be your dad.

P.S. Tell Casey (the big dog) that I will send him a letter as soon as possible.

Magnatron Doolittle, Ms. Meghan Marre, "the most beautiful 6-year-old girl in the world."

Tell Mom, "Hey Baby, What's shakin?" Give her a bear hug for me.

Love,
Dad

Our worlds became condensed to sporadic visits, written letters, and calls from a landline. None of us had cell phones at that time. There was no Facebook to post news or pictures. We used the resources we had to stay in touch the best we could. It was so hard to be apart.

Once, as the sole caregiver for Logan, I got sick and couldn't take care of him very well. Our friend Gary picked him up for his clinic appointments, and Logan took care of me. The rules at RMH included no children in the kitchen unsupervised. Logan was ten, and we had no choice, so he cooked meals for the two of us. The other residents of the house quickly realized Logan was mature and capable despite his age.

Eight

SPECIAL TIMES

For twenty months, we spent holidays and birthdays either in the hospital or at Ronald McDonald House. One of the kids' favorite holidays was Halloween. They loved to go trick-or-treating. The co-owner of E. J. Bartells, Erik Jensen, picked Casey and Meghan up on Halloween and took them to load up on candy. Logan and I participated in Children's Hospital's Halloween activities. He was disappointed that he couldn't wear a costume because of all the tubes he had in him. The hospital was good about providing activities for the kids, so they didn't feel too sad about being there. We had a good time, and Logan decorated his room with gifts from friends and family. I still have those decorations, and every Halloween I pull them out and remember the fun evening the two of us shared. Despite the dreariness of being in a hospital, we tried to have as much fun as we could.

I loved climbing into bed with Logan and watching *Scooby Doo* with him. We would take walks all around the hospital. He loved playing pranks on his nurses and doctors. One day, a doctor he didn't particularly like, came into his room. Logan asked him if he had ever tried a Warhead. The doctor told him he hadn't, so Logan convinced him he must try one. We took a walk around the unit, and Logan kept watching the doctor's face as we went by. When he saw the grim look due to the sour candy, he burst out laughing. He cracked himself up. Another time he had Flarp, a slimy "noise putty" that made a sound as if he was passing gas when he put his finger in it. He had it under the sheet and kept doing it when a nurse was changing his IV bag. She exclaimed, "Logan!" and he laughed and laughed. There were not too many dull moments when mischievous Logan was in the building.

My parents, Casey, and Meghan flew back and forth many times to visit us. Sometimes my parents traded off with us and became the caregivers so we could spend time with Casey and Meghan. We tried to normalize everything as best we could. One time, Dad flew in to surprise Logan in the hospital. He dressed up as Dr. Cueball, a character he invented, and brought Logan homemade bread from Granny. Dad wore a big plastic nose, a beard, and glasses. He really fooled Logan. Logan was ecstatic to see his Pockie, but he was also excited about his bread. Logan did *not* want to share that bread. He was a generous soul but stingy if it involved Granny's bread.

One special incident comes to mind when I think about our time together. Logan felt well enough to go out, and we went to McDonald's. He put Meghan on his lap and force-fed her a french fry. It was a delightful and normal time! He was feeling a bit guilty because a few days before that, he had been grumpy (due to the steroids affecting his moods) and had gotten mad at Meghan and told her she was a "mistake." He was referring to my pregnancy with her after the vasectomy Patrick had before she was born. He felt so bad about that and tried to make it up to her. The steroids really affected his moods, and he tried to keep that in mind when he got moody, but sometimes things got the better of him.

One sunny day, Patrick and I took Logan to the Woodland Park Zoo in Seattle. We were having so much fun just walking around with him. We walked by a couple of kangaroos mating. Logan said, "Not in front of the children!" He was as quick-witted as his father.

Besides being witty, Logan was also very kind to younger children. There were a couple of very young children at Ronald McDonald House. Zoey was about eighteen months old when she was diagnosed with ALL. She needed to learn to swallow adult-size pills. Logan taught her how to do so, and she wouldn't take her pills unless Logan or Casey would sit next to her. Lake and Ariel would follow Logan all around the house, and Shelby would just plop on his lap.

One night all of us parents cranked up the music and danced around the house with our sick kids. We were all so happy because they were alive and not in the hospital. I especially remember little Jordan singing "Walking around the Sun" at the top of her lungs. All these years later, I remember the joy on her precious little face. Jordan didn't survive long after that day, but that night, the sheer joy she felt radiated on her and through her and was tangible to us all.

Before we came home on December 12, 1997, we got to go on a Christmas cruise with Casey and Meghan. They took us to the boat by limo. The kids were thoroughly impressed, and we had a fabulous time with other families from Ronald McDonald House. I embarrassed Logan because I was dancing with a bunch of the other mothers. He didn't like his mom dancing at all unless it was with his dad.

One nice thing about RMH was that we were often given opportunities to attend events to normalize our situation. Logan got to go to many Mariners' games, the circus, the zoo, and many other fabulous events. We appreciated the efforts of so many who tried to make things easier.

Once I confided with a friend from church that we felt lonely and were missing home. She told the pastor, who shared it with our congregation. They decided to make a video for Logan. In it, everyone in church rose to his or her feet and clapped and shouted, "Logan, Logan, Logan," repeatedly. To this day, my eyes fill with tears for the joy and the relief Logan felt realizing he had not been forgotten and that people were continuing to pray for him and support him.

Logan became famous in our community even while we were away. There were stories written about him in both our Valley and Anchorage newspapers. He even made the TV news! He got many cards and presents sent to him, which made him so happy. Several people ran marathons for the Leukemia & Lymphoma Society in his honor. Logan planned to run a marathon when he was better, so he could raise money for the LLS. It was important to him that a cure for all cancers would be found.

Logan loved being a celebrity and willingly gave interviews. All who knew him loved him, and he ate up the attention like a cat licking cream out of a bowl. He threw himself into rebuilding his strength and stamina. He was determined to beat this horrific insult to his health.

Logan was selected to be an Iditarod Rider for the Make-A-Wish Foundation. He got to ride with Jeff King, a well-known Iditarod champion, in his dogsled, at the start of the Iditarod 1998. He was recognized and honored at the Iditarod banquet. Cabela's sponsored the Make-A-Wish event, and Logan got outfitted with many cool things from their outdoor-recreation store. He also got to make a commercial for Make-A-Wish with Jeff King. There were so many "takes" in making the commercial, and we cracked up as we caught Logan rolling his eyes as he was told to emphasize a different word each take. Finally, there was success. Later we learned that the TV station wasn't going to air the commercial because of one error stating how many times Jeff King had won the Iditarod race. We were sincerely disappointed. Later, Logan's video was aired at a large celebration to honor him. Our boy was, and continues to be, a superstar.

Nine

WARNING SIGNS FOLLOWED BY DISAPPOINTMENT

Things were going well until April of 1998. On April 13, his blood work showed his platelets were down to 36,000. Normal is above 150,000. The doctors took him off chemo. On April 16, Dr. Keller examined him and discovered his spleen was enlarged. On the eighteenth, his platelets were down to 27,000. While in Providence Hospital, we ran into my cousin Matt and his wife, Mary. They were there to welcome the birth of their firstborn child while we were mourning the apparent relapse of our firstborn. On April 20, we headed back to Seattle.

Logan had the usual blood tests at Children's Hospital. The receptionist had Logan's labs pulled up on the computer, and I saw them when I went to ask her a question. I could see that they had found blasts cells in his blood. Although in my heart I already knew he had relapsed, it still hit me like a ton of bricks falling on my chest and crushing me. Hadn't he been through enough? We had fought as hard as we could. We had taken him to a fabulous hospital. We had believed he would be okay. This was supposed to be the "good leukemia." Why?

We were told he had to get a bone marrow transplant to survive. We held out hope that one of us would be a match. At the time, a simple blood test was done to test for a match. Unfortunately, none of us matched Logan, but ironically, Casey and Meghan were identical matches for each other. A national search was done, and there was not one single person on the registry who matched our boy. Now we knew Logan was special, but this was ridiculous. A match had to be found quickly so our boy could be cured.

Soon, I was alone with Logan again and trying to cope the best I could. One day, while receiving a blood transfusion, Logan had a craving for Taco Bell. I drove to pick it up and ended up getting a parking ticket because I didn't realize I had parked in a loading zone. I called Patrick from a pay phone hysterically crying because I was worried about the extra cost I had caused. He was quick to reassure me that it was going to be okay. I found myself going from a positive attitude to hysteria from time to time as I coped with my son's serious illness.

We started all over again, trying to make him better by infusing the poison in his bloodstream. Would it work? Would our brave boy reach remission again? Per our doctors, chemotherapy wouldn't be enough. If the cancer came back once, it would come back again.

On the fourth of July, we were told Logan's only option was to receive an unrelated umbilical cord stem-cell transplant. At that time, only around five hundred of these transplants had been done. A cord-blood transplant involves using the stem cells of the umbilical cord that a baby's parents donated to a national cord bank after birth. We were frightened beyond belief, but filled with hope.

Killing Leuk

Logan had to go through a lot of testing, along with intense chemo and radiation, before his transplant. He went from doctor to doctor getting his eyes, teeth, ears, and mind examined. Yes, our smart boy had to get an IQ test as well. They discovered what we already knew: he was highly intelligent. We had a lot of fun going to each of his appointments, and I chronicled his journey, snapping pictures at each "station."

By this time, Logan was being treated at the Fred Hutchinson Cancer Research Center in Seattle rather than at Children's Hospital. Once again Logan was surrounded by children in the waiting room. The little ones were always drawn to him. One day, several little kids surrounded him and wanted him to play "Ring-around-the Rosie." He did so without complaint, but I could tell he was tired.

The radiation was the worst part of pretransplant preparation. Logan bravely entered the room and endured three days of it. He came out of the sessions with migraines and vomiting. Despite his obvious discomfort, he did his best to remain positive and happy.

The day we had prepared for arrived. We didn't know what to expect and found the actual "transplant" to be uneventful. The lifesaving stem cells were hung in a plastic bag on his IV pole, just like his many blood transfusions. The process was completed in about twenty minutes. The stem cells smelled like creamed corn, which was gross. Logan chose to listen to "Fuel" by Metallica as he welcomed his lifesaving stem cells. "Gimme fuel, Gimme fire, Gimme that which I desire." Not my kind of music, but this was ALL about Logan! Afterward, we stayed in the hospital for a few weeks.

During this time, Logan suffered from terrible mouth sores, body aches, and a loss of appetite. Despite all of that, he was positive and hopeful and continued to charm his doctors and nurses. Each day I would write what day it was and how he felt that day. Transplant day was Day Zero, and the succeeding days were Day One, Day Two, and so forth. Logan would assess how he felt each day and make sure he said the right descriptive adjective. He was always positive and would say he felt terrific even when it was obvious he didn't. He would think carefully how to express how he felt. I have one picture showing that he originally chose "good" to describe how he felt and then asked me to draw a line through it and had me write "awesome." The poor kid found it very difficult to talk with all those mouth sores, but we found a way to communicate.

His transplant took place at Swedish Hospital. They had a neat meal program, and Logan could order whatever food he wanted whenever he wanted it. I encouraged him to try all sorts of things, but he just wasn't hungry. When he was finally released back to our apartment, his first choice of meal was tuna noodle casserole and strawberries. I had never been so excited to cook a meal before. Unfortunately, he just couldn't eat it. It always seemed as though we were taking one step forward and two steps back.

Taking care of Logan away from the hospital was a little nerve-racking. I was responsible for making sure he got plenty of rest and wasn't exposed to sick people. One night we were invited over to Dr. Frangoul's house for dinner. I had to call him and tell him Logan wasn't feeling well. He was urinating blood. Dr. Frangoul said we needed to go to the emergency room right away. It seemed so often that Logan ended up in the emergency room while the TV show *ER* was on. We laughed about it through our tears of disappointment.

On September 26, I made note that Logan had a temperature of 102, and they didn't know what was wrong. Dad came down from Alaska to help me, and I went back to the apartment to sleep for a bit. Logan received platelets, but his count actually went down instead of up. He was still urinating blood. He was having trouble breathing and was receiving respiratory treatments.

Ten

SERIOUS COMPLICATIONS

*T*he following are excerpts from the e-mail notifications I sent daily to friends and family:

September 28, 1998: Logan's condition has not improved. He has a temperature of 103.3. His pulse is 156 beats per minute. All the respiratory tests they have done have come back negative. The chest x-ray shows something, but they are not sure what. One minute they are telling us he will probably be discharged today, and the next minute he's having trouble breathing and his temperature shoots up. It's the minute-by-minute thing that gets to me! It's a violent roller coaster ride. We were told that Logan has parainfluenza 3 and it should get better on its own. But wait, now we are told he must have a CT scan because they suspect the virus is further down then they thought. I was told they may have to put him under general anesthesia and do a wash with a scope. If it shows positive, he'll have to do all sorts of treatments. They'll consider releasing him on Wednesday. He is in strict isolation. No one can come in unless they are gowned and masked including eye gear. Dad and I can't leave the room unless we put on the whole outfit outside his room. Once again everything is uncertain. It's very frustrating, but we'll just trust the Lord to do all the worrying for us.

September 29, 1998: The pulmonary doctors strongly feel Logan has pneumonia. This is a fear I had all along. I know a little girl who came through the transplant just fine, then got pneumonia and died. I'm a little nervous to say the least.

September 30, 1998: We still don't know for sure, but the doctors told us to prepare for the worst. He could very well die from this. They think it's a fungal infection. He is in a lot of pain physically and emotionally. He is going in for a lung biopsy at 2:00 p.m. They couldn't tell us anything from yesterday's testing. Patrick is coming in at two o'clock, and someone from E. J. Bartells will pick him up and bring him to the hospital. Logan is on oxygen because he's having trouble breathing. He still has a fever. He cried all night because he couldn't urinate. They inserted a catheter. He has a virus called BK virus, which caused him to urinate blood. A clot has formed near the opening of his bladder, and no urine could come out. The catheter came out while he was peeing after receiving medication to relax his bladder. They did his first ribavirin treatment. He must be in a tent, and only one person can be with him. Dad has been taking the honors, and he must totally gown and mask up. He is taking an antifungal called Amphoterian B. It can cause high fevers and chills.

September 30, 1998: They postponed the lung biopsy till 3:30, and Patrick got here just in time. God's timing. They let me go in while they did the procedure. They got two good vials of fluid. Hopefully they'll be up with results soon. They said the culture from yesterday's bronchoscopy came back positive for parainfluenza 3. I think that's good news, but the doctors are still saying they don't think that's why there are lumps on his lungs. There is a nodule on each lung. They still think it's a fungal infection. They tell us there is minimal chance of treating a fungal infection. He will get ribavirin three times a day for seven days. I believe each treatment is for two hours. He will also be getting immunoglobin shots to raise his white blood count. His ANC dropped to 460 today.

I don't want to call anyone because whenever I hear someone's voice, I start bawling, and it upsets Logan. We feel surrounded by the Lord's presence. We have had many people praying for Logan. We ask you to increase the numbers and add even more prayers to the list. Logan's organs have remained strong through this, and we know we've come too far to let something bad happen to him now. We feel he is strong enough physically, spiritually, and emotionally to fight this thing and win the battle. I'm not saying we aren't nervous, upset, or scared. We are all the above and more. But...we are also Christians with great faith. Please pray specifically for Logan's healing. God hears our prayers and our cries to heaven. Also, please pray for the other children and adults who are afflicted with this horrible disease. It's not an easy life to lead.

October 1, 1998: The doctors came in and said the results won't be back until tomorrow. They are having a surgeon from Children's Hospital come to review the reports. He is having his third biopsy of the week. They keep telling us to expect the worst. They repaired his lumen today. We need both sides for his growing number of medications. He seems much better today, and his pulse is just about normal. He got off oxygen this morning but later had to go back on it. His catheter has clogged, and he's uncomfortable. We're mentally exhausted. This waiting game is so hard. I don't know how many times I can hear "We don't know yet" before I scream at the doctors. I know it's not their fault, but it is so hard on us.

October 2, 1998: Franci came by to visit. It was so comforting to have her here. Logan was sleeping the whole time. His fever is going back up. Last check showed it was 101. He's pretty sick today. Yesterday, late afternoon and evening were horrible. He was in so much discomfort with the catheter. He was like a woman in labor, panting and pushing as hard as he could while squeezing my hand. He kept thinking if he pushed, the clot would come out. It was heartbreaking. The surgeon came in and described how today's biopsy will be, and Logan became very upset. He is sick of hearing about it all. He is terrified. Last night was a real emotional drain for us. His ANC is up to 1,300 today, thanks to the GCFS shots. His urine is clear today, so hopefully that means an end to the pain and discomfort.

Please pray that when they do the biopsy that they won't find any nodules. I've heard of such miracles before, and I totally believe God can do this. If we all stand together and ask, maybe He'll answer our prayer in the way we want Him to. Wouldn't this be a totally awesome God-given miracle? Logan has a fever, and he doesn't want anyone to touch him. It makes it hard on me, breaks my heart actually. I want to hold him and kiss him, but he doesn't want me near. I suppose I wouldn't want anyone near me either if I felt as bad as he does. I'm feeling a little sorry for myself. I don't have any children to hold right now, and I don't even have a dog to pet. It's been seven weeks since I have seen Casey and Meghan, and I miss them so much. They also found strep in the culture, so he has that on top of the parainfluenza 3. Logan has a hard road ahead. I know you are praying faithfully, and we are so very, very grateful. We must not stop though.

The surgery took three hours including recovery time. The surgery was successful! They believe they removed the whole nodule on the right lung. We don't know the results of that yet. They also found the lining of his lung stuck to his chest wall. They peeled it back and found pus there. They took a swab of that and sent it to the lab. We have no idea when we will find out the results. He came through it all okay but is in a lot of pain. He has a tube sticking out of his chest, which maintains negative pleural pressure so his lung won't collapse. That will need to stay in place for two to three days depending on how they think his lung is doing. While in surgery, they used the lumen they repaired yesterday with no problem. By the time he was in recovery, it had stopped working again!

Now they are talking about putting an IV in his hand. I am furious. I have about had it with all the things they are doing to my child. They don't seem to want to call someone more qualified and experienced to fix the problem. I had a heated conversation with the doctor on call and "persuaded" her to call someone who can help. If I have to, I will call Dr. Hickman himself. He's the one that put the Hickman line in and the one they named it after. I don't think these people have children, because if they did, they would be a little more compassionate.

Before his surgery, the anesthesiologist came up and asked us the usual questions before anesthesia, such as "Does Logan have any allergies? Has he had any problems with *anesthesia, and has any family member had a problem with anesthesia?" We answered no to all the questions. All of a sudden Logan piped up and said, "Well, actually in our family we do have problems with anesthesia." The doctor asked, "What kind of problems, Logan?" Logan replied, "We all fall asleep!" The doctor loved that. He is so quick-witted.*

Logan is now watching *Dirty Harry* and chewing bubble gum. He's waiting for Pockie to bring him the movie *Titanic*. They agreed to skip his ribavirin treatment tonight, and Logan is relieved not to be under the tent.

Eleven

The Worst News

*C*ontinued *excerpts I sent to friends and family.*

October 3, 1998: The doctors came in this morning and told us the pathologist reported it is definitely a fungal infection. Obviously, it's not the diagnosis we wanted. We have a couple of good things going for us: They think they got all the fungus on the right side, and his lungs aren't too diminished. They feel good about the amount of oxygen he is consuming. His liver functions are up, and his bilirubin is high. His eyes are jaundiced. They don't know why that is happening right now. Right now, they aren't too concerned, but it could mean a biopsy at a later point. His condition is serious but stable. Our hearts are heavy. We ask for your continued prayers. This is our special little boy. We love him so much.

October 6, 1998: The doctors came in this morning and gave us the news. It is Aspergillus, the worst kind of fungal infection to have. They will probably do another CT scan today and will be scheduling surgery to remove the other nodule. They will probably add another antibiotic too. The amphotericin they have him on can damage his kidneys. His kidney functions are already high. His ANC is up to 1600, and they are tapering him off steroids. With steroids being out of the picture and his white blood counts going up, he has a better chance for survival. He had another high fever last night and was up the whole night. He's having pain in his side again, and now his abdomen is tender to touch. Pray for a complete healing and peace for him. He's very anxious.

Here's an update to this morning's report: He's fever-free and starting to recover from the last three surgeries and isn't as afraid to move. He will be having his fourth surgery this week, tomorrow. They will be removing the nodule on his left lung. There has been concern as to whether they'll be able to remove it. From the CT scan, it appears the lump may be attached to his aorta, but it may be just beside it. They don't think they can remove it if it's attached. The surgeon came in this morning and seemed confident he can remove it. Please pray for guidance with the surgeon that the nodule can be easily removed, and his lungs will not collapse, and they will get it all. The CT scan showed some swelling in his abdomen. He's been complaining of pain in his side the past three weeks. The doctors kept telling him it was muscular. I never thought so, but they wouldn't do anything about it. Now they say it's inflamed, and they are withholding all food and drink for a limited time to give his bowels a rest. They are also switching antibiotics in hopes of getting rid of these fevers that are there every day.

His breathing is still labored, and his heart rate was 171 this morning at rest. His SAT was 90 percent while on the oxygen and 85-87 percent when off. His body is still consuming platelets quickly. He gets platelet transfusions every day. Amazingly, his hematocrit (red blood cells) held on for quite some time. His ANC was up to 1630 today. The doctors are pleased with the tapering of the steroids. He can fight this much better being off them.

October 7, 1998: Logan is out of surgery and is doing okay. He's in a lot of pain and moaning in his sleep a lot. We're getting a PCA pump in here so he can self-inject morphine when he needs it. His SAT is 97 percent with oxygen. The surgery was successful. They were able to remove the nodule. It was in the lining of his aorta, but they could remove it with the scope rather than the open lung procedure. They made four incisions instead of three like they did on the other side. He has a chest tube in again, but hopefully they can take that out tomorrow. Chest x-rays show his lungs are expanding well. Now we just wait for the results of the cultures. I don't think the treatment will change at all. They decided against the other antifungal drug because they have been known to counteract each other.

We have a new problem that has developed. His abdomen is distended and very painful to touch. They've thrown out a whole bunch of possibilities, but basically, they don't have any idea. I've seen many children whose stomachs are swollen like this, and the outcome wasn't good. It is a scary thing. We think we can beat one odd thing and then we get hit with another one. We're still praying hard for a miracle and an end to these problems. I have a sign on the door that says "GOD IS THE GREAT PHYSICIAN." I tell everyone who comes in to enter with a prayerful attitude. I ask the medical staff to pray for guidance to do the right thing for Logan.

Allen and Kathy Conn flew down to be with us. What a blessing to have them there. We prayed for Logan before surgery, and they have been praying for him all afternoon. We know how many are praying, and we are comforted. We really appreciate our church family for standing behind us and beside us. They have faithfully prayed for Logan and our family. Dr. Martin (our family physician in Alaska) came to see Logan too since he was in Seattle for a conference.

I read a sheet on Aspergillus statistics. There is a 7 percent success rate. If the patient makes it two weeks, the success rate goes up to 33 percent. God is bigger than a statistic. Plus, Logan is not a statistic! He is Logan, our special, special boy. He still has fevers, and they don't know why. Thank you for your prayers. You have blessed our lives. Thank you for sharing your stories of how Logan has blessed your lives.

October 8, 1998: Last night around seven o'clock, Logan started feeling awesome. He was happy and elated. His fever was gone, and he was on cloud nine. About five o'clock this morning, Patrick called me and panicked. Logan's resting pulse was over 200, and his blood pressure was up, and he was having trouble breathing.

Kelly Marre

The oxygen wasn't helping him much. Patrick told me I needed to come right away. I grabbed the kids, yelled at mom, and we got to the hospital in less than ten minutes. When we walked in, everything was in control. His fever was 103, and they were thinking that's what caused the problems. They did a chest x-ray, and his lung was not collapsed. I can't describe the feelings of fear. I just locked myself in the bathroom for a while until I calmed down. I cried hysterically, and my heart was pounding. I felt physically sick. I thought this was it. He better never scare me like that again!

Right now he's feeling better. He is being really sweet to all of us. He has wanted his brother and sister around constantly. Meghan is in bed with him right now. He insisted she lie beside him. She was more than willing to do this. Casey and Meghan love Logan so much and are so worried about him. Casey just read Logan a card he got in the mail, and Meghan read the other card to him. They are the neatest kids. They are so caring. This never seems to make them feel left out or resentful. They just focus on their brother.

His ANC is 2,270 today! Praise God for that! We have had doctors, surgeons, infectious-disease control, nurses, and others in here this morning, and all seem pretty positive. They are all amazed how well he is doing and how little he complains. He is quite the champion.

His stomach is even more swollen today. They think he might have a touch of air in there from the surgeries and the oxygen. We are trying to coach him into belching. Can you believe it? Maybe he and Casey can have a contest on who can burp the loudest. Casey would love it for sure.

I know your prayers will continue. Please pray especially for his counts to continue going up, stomach to go down, and fevers to break. The doctors say it's possible that there is more fungus in his body, but they just can't see it at this time. Please pray they are wrong.

Killing Leuk

October 9, 1998: Well, my friends, if you believe in miracles, pray for them now. The doctors say the only thing that will save our son is a miracle from God. They can't do anything else. They are not stopping the treatments, but it's apparent they are not working. They got the report back today. The fungal infection has infiltrated through his lungs, vessels, and other parts. They say he has three to five days left. We are heartbroken, angry, and sad. We're still holding on to hope. When the doctors told us, I ran from the room and wrapped my arms around Logan. He kept asking me what was wrong, and I couldn't tell him. I don't want him scared.

If we don't have hope, what do we have? Right now he's doing well and is playing poker with his visitors. We have lots of family coming in tomorrow. Granny, Pockie, Grandma Michele, Uncle Mark, Aunt Sharmin, Michelle, Melissa, Holly, Uncle Mike, Aunt Linda, Jessica, and Nick.

We haven't told him. We are still encouraging him to beat this thing. We are trying to make this a fun week for him. The doctors want us to sign a "do not resuscitate" form. That is like taking a stake and ramming it into my heart. How could this happen? Why my good, wonderful son who would never hurt anyone?

We pray for strength, for understanding, for continued hope. We ask God to comfort us to help us through this. Pray for a miracle; we believe in miracles.

October 11, 1998: Logan had an awesome day today. He played Nintendo for about three hours. He held his new baby cousin, burped her, and admired her. I wish you could see the sparkle in his eyes when he looks at her. It's precious. He is thrilled to have his whole family here. He doesn't like it when anyone leaves the room. He enjoys the noise.

His ANC is over 3,000 today! He lost a few ounces of fluid that he's been retaining. He slept all night with no fevers or problems. It was awesome. Patrick and I got some sleep too. We were able to turn his oxygen down to 40 percent a while ago. This morning it was up to 90 percent.

Logan stood up for quite a while and did some easy stretching exercises. He thought that felt really good. Last night he got a surprise visit from his good buddy Josh Saxon. His eyes lit up because he's so happy. My heart was so touched when I heard Josh pray with Logan.

We had two guys come and sing for Logan today. We enjoyed having them. We believe in miracles. We continue praying for one. Things are looking a little positive right now, and we pray it continues to be positive. We started him on an herbal product last night. He gets it every four hours. They crush it up and put it in his NG tube.

We are having a surprise birthday party for Meghan today. Her birthday is actually Friday, but we want to have it while everyone is here and Logan is feeling good. When you pray, BELIEVE that God can and will heal Logan. I do NOT want any doubts. Let's stand together and BELIEVE.

October 12, 1998: Last night Logan wanted to play Uno. We played two hands. He won one, and Pockie won the other. It was a great time. We cranked up his Elvis CD and partied. Most of his family left last night and today. Aunt Suzanne is still here. Granny and Grandpa are here until tomorrow, and my parents are still here. His friend Alex VonWalter is coming to visit him today.

The doctors came in this morning and admitted he's doing better than they thought he was. They're cautious, but how can they not see this as healing? I want us all to agree together that God will and can heal Logan. His kidney and liver functions are elevated, yet not too much. He had a really bad fever this morning. He's still battling it, but he's better. He has been drinking Pepsi today (not something I normally let him do)! His NG tube is clogged; maybe from the herbs. We're not sure what we are going to do about that. His abdomen is terribly swollen, but they say it's fluid, and they think it will go down. His ANC dropped to 2,700 today, but that's still a good number. Let's pray it goes to over 5,000. That would be great! I appreciate all your positive e-mails. I don't want ANYONE to have doubts. Our God is an awesome God. Logan has touched so many lives.

The social worker came in to talk with me. She is really pushing us to tell Logan the truth—that they think he's going to die. I can't do that. I can't tell him that. I don't want our baby to be scared. I deliberately stayed on the phone when she came in the room. I know it was rude, but I didn't want to talk to her.

October 13, 1998: I apologize for the late update. Logan was having such an awesome day, and I couldn't tear myself away from the Uno games, the Monopoly game, and just visiting with him. I felt sorry for him, so I sold him a property in Monopoly. Then when I landed on it, he kept making me pay. I was eventually bankrupt. I said, "But Logan, we are family!" He said, "Business is business."

Now I'm about to fall asleep. It's 10:30 p.m., and we're watching movies. This morning Logan woke up with a 104-degree fever, but it didn't last past noon, thank goodness. Even through the fever, he was visiting with his friend Alex and playing Nintendo. They had a really nice visit.

He has had a couple new things come up. One is a weird ring around his belly button. It appears to be growing a little. They're not really sure what it is but feel it's some sort of infection, maybe staph. His lungs sound about the same, and the air pockets around the lungs are reabsorbing. One doctor thought his lungs sounded a little better today. We are confident tomorrow they'll really notice a difference. He got up and did some more knee bends, arm raises, and walking in place. He sat in a chair while I read to him. We are reading the Goose Bumps series. This particular book is The Boy Who Learned to Fly.

We had lots of visitors again today, but he drew the limit and kicked everyone but family out. He's really tired. He stayed awake most of the day. He only slept about ten minutes. He is used to sleeping four to eight hours during the day, so I think he's just worn out. We are excited that Logan's friend Kekoa Davis will be coming to see him

Thursday. He really enjoyed Josh and Alex's visits. It means a lot to him and all of us to have the support. We really appreciate the Conns being here with us. They've been a comforting presence. We appreciate our church and their desire to help.

We cannot tell you how much we appreciate your support. Your prayers and beliefs in the miracle of Logan's healing are so appreciated. Thank you for standing with us before God and praising Him for all the good He has done. Our God is an awesome God. We believe God is doing a miracle in Logan.

Twelve

ROLLER COASTER

*A*gain, I think excerpts from my e-mail updates best capture our mood and wildly swinging emotions as we waited to see if Logan would turn the corner.

October 14, 1998: Here we go again. Another roller coaster ride, and it's not a smooth sailing, bump-free ride. I've never imagined my emotions can change so quickly from one second to another. The only thing that stays constant is in my Lord's ability to heal Logan. Our prayers don't change; we pray for complete healing.

The middle of the night started with another bad fever. It goes up to 104 most mornings but usually disappears by noon. Today it lasted all day until 7:00 p.m. He pretty much slept till 4:00 p.m. The doctor came in and told us his chest x-ray is worse. She saw stripes on his lungs, which they feel is Aspergillus. We were crushed. For one moment, we felt defeated, but then we refused to feel that way. God is in control, and we are not going to stop our prayers for a miracle. We refuse to be defeated. We refuse to give up. Logan refuses to give up. When he woke up and the fever started going away, he asked his visitors to come into the room and play Uno with him. We played five hands. What an elated time it is when he feels good!

The rough ride is killing us. Our bodies cannot take much more of the stress. High one moment, low the next. How much more can we take? The kids are brought to tears easily. They're not eating like they should, and they won't leave often. It's not healthy for them to continuously be in here. I'm trying to talk them into going out a little bit each day. They love their brother so much.

Granny, Grandpa Bill, and Aunt Suzanne left this morning. My friends Stacey and Allen and Kathy are leaving tomorrow. That leaves Pockie, Grandma, and us. Kekoa will arrive in the morning. Logan will be thrilled. He is getting overwhelmed with the many people who have come to visit. He wouldn't let anyone in his room until this evening. He just felt so bad. His stomach seems to be getting more swollen. It is shocking to see his poor battered body. It's amazing someone with so many physical problems can continue to want to play games and visit.

Logan put me in charge of giving him his growth factor shots. They make his ANC go up. He didn't like the way some of the shots felt, so he decided I could give better ones. Tonight was the third night I did it. He says he doesn't even feel it when I give it to him. Thank God! It's hard for me to do it. I pray before I put it in that I won't hurt him and that tomorrow's counts will be even higher.

Today's ANC was 2,600. He got platelets and red blood today. They've also started giving him vancomycin, the drug he had during transplant. It had caused "red man syndrome," but he didn't seem to have any problems with it today. As always, we are grateful for your prayers for a miracle. We still believe in one with all our hearts.

October 15, 1998: Last night Logan did not have a fever. He's still fever-free today, praise God! He feels so much better when he doesn't have that to worry about. Breathing is harder for him. We had to increase his oxygen up to 45 percent. The doctors came in this morning and feel he's worse. They don't hear breath sounds down low anymore. He's only using the top half of his lungs. His neck muscles move constantly with the struggle to breathe.

He doesn't feel bad, doesn't feel great. Just not in the mood to do push-ups or run long miles. Right now, he is watching a movie with Casey and Meghan. We're hanging in there. Praying for that miracle...Please don't stop praying and believing in the miracle Logan needs. We need you all to beg God for it. We have faith. We know God can provide it. Pray He hears our cries.

October 16, 1998: Last night brought us another restless night. Logan had a low-grade fever all night. He talks in his sleep constantly and thrashes about. It makes us all worn out. This morning we were relieved not to have a fever for once. It didn't kick in until this afternoon, when it shot up to 103. Unfortunately, he slept all morning. He seems so tired. He's been awake off and on since this afternoon. He slept through most of Meghan's birthday party.

The doctors came in this morning and cautiously told me that Logan is "holding his own." His oxygen rate remains at 45 percent. His chest x-rays are the same as Wednesday's. His stomach MIGHT be a little smaller. The redness on his belly button is getting a little better. They even mentioned testing him again in one or two weeks for parainfluenza. You realize what this means, right? They must be getting confident! I know WE are.

His NG tube clogged. They have tried everything and can't get it unclogged. We have to get another one. This poor baby. The nurse told him she couldn't get anything in or out. He very quietly said, "I know." She told him she would have to put in another one. He spoke so gently when he said, "That's okay." They do it awake. For those of you who don't know, it's a tube that goes up his nose, down his throat, and into his abdomen.

Then I had to tell him to pick a spot for his shot. He said, "Okay, right here." I don't know which is harder on me: him being so used to everything and continuing to say please and thank you, or when he cries in pain. All I know is he is my hero and my champion, and I am so very proud of him. He is an awesome child, and I thank God for him every moment.

Today is Meghan's seventh birthday. She enjoyed her party. Grandma made her a kitty cake. She got lots of presents, and it was a special day for her. She wanted to know where the candles for her cake were. I explained that she couldn't have candles because of Logan's oxygen. She said, "Oh, that's okay, I don't mind." Logan was almost in tears because he felt so guilty. There was no need; she only wanted her brother. Gary Moffat bought her a Spice Girls CD. She danced and sang until Logan was about to kick her out. We had many from E. J. Bartells come to celebrate with us. They are some of the neatest people anyone could ever meet. When all our relatives came, they took turns chauffeuring between here, the airport, and their houses, where everyone stayed. They spent last weekend helping us through the crisis and brought us food. Today they held a special prayer for Logan in their office.

Aunt Connie and Uncle Mike have a brief layover, so they are going to come see Logan. Our friends Travis and Beth came by today on their layover. It's wonderful to see familiar faces. In times of trouble, it's good to know we have so many friends. What's even nicer is hearing people say they are praying for Logan and mean it. I know you are faithfully praying. God hears your prayers.

October 17, 1998: How should I title this page? Answers to prayers are taking place? Christians be encouraged—God is doing great things in Logan? Happy Day?

Are you ready for our news? Logan's ANC is over 5,000 today! His white blood count is 6,000, and his stomach is smaller today. He hasn't had Tylenol all day today, and his fever is going down. Right now, it's 101. He played ball this morning. We had a game of hot potato going on. Now he's playing his fourth hand of Uno. He, Kekoa, and my mom are playing.

The doctors came in this morning and said they were encouraged. Logan is surprising them. We're not surprised; we have never lost our faith in God's ability to heal Logan. We are a long way from total health, but we feel really positive about it. He had to have his oxygen rate increased this morning because his resting pulse was 160. They increased it to 60 percent. We are hoping we will be able to turn it back down when his fever goes away.

Last night Logan slept in his chair all night! His choice, really. Patrick and I took his hospital bed. Casey and Kekoa each had a cot here in the room. Meghan slept in the dayroom with my parents. I never thought I could live in a twenty-by-twelve room with so many people and sharing only one bathroom. But hey, we are doing it well! It's amazing how much we can do when we have to. We need you to pray as hard as you have been. God IS doing great things, but we have a long way to go and really need this miracle. It will be a great witness to so many unbelievers to have Logan healed. Thank you for all your encouraging messages and powerful prayers.

October 18, 1998: Well, today is definitely not as good of a day as yesterday. Logan is fevering. He had been really sleepy and can't seem to stay awake today. This morning he was having a very hard time breathing. They had to increase his oxygen to 70 percent. They have since put it back down to 60 percent. His fever is close to 103. Logan's friend Kameron, from RMH, is here visiting with him. They are trying to play Nintendo, but Logan keeps falling asleep. It's great entertainment for Casey to have Kameron here. Hopefully Logan will turn around here soon and will be up to playing.

His ANC dropped down to 4,500 this morning. We'll see how it looks tomorrow. We might have to go back on the GCSF shots to keep it up there. Chest x-rays and abdomen x-rays look the same. No news is good news, right? We now have him on colloidal silver.

October 19, 1998: Last night was a pretty good night for Logan. He slept pretty well and didn't start fevering until about four o'clock this morning. He took some Tylenol, and it's down to ninety-nine. We no longer give him Tylenol around the clock, and his liver functions are a little better. His oxygen is still at 60 percent. He's sleeping right now and seems to be breathing better. His color looks really good. He was wide awake earlier and quite alert. We have been having him stand up and go to the bathroom instead of just lying there. This way he's getting a little exercise and expanding his lungs more. He's been working his spirometer and getting it up to almost five hundred. I'm alternating between the colloidal silver and a cream from the Awareness Herbal Company on his belly, and it's getting a lot better. It's quite challenging to do these herbs. I don't want to leave his NG unclamped for too long.

The doctors say his lungs sound about the same this morning. They even said they want to do another CT scan in a couple of days and possibly remove his NG tube. They said they don't want to give us false hope, but he's certainly holding his own. They won't make promises, but they're being more positive. At least I take that as positive! I think they are really surprised he is still here and doing pretty well. His ANC is 5,350 today, and that's without the shots! His white blood count is 6,770, which is good.

Kameron spent the night in the room with us last night. Logan likes having a buddy around. We went to bed after midnight again. We're keeping terrible hours around here. Patrick hardly sleeps the night at all. He naps during the day when he can. I don't hear at night as well as he does. If Logan moves an inch, he jumps up. He is such an awesome father. It's taken all of us to do this. We're quite comical at times, and we each have a role and a job. Right now, Mom is doing the housekeeper's job. She is cleaning the trash can and moving furniture around. I think she is bored. Keep the prayers coming!

Evening update: Logan had a great day. He only needed Tylenol three times today. His fever got up to 102. It doesn't seem to last as long, and the fevers are getting fewer in between. Praise God! He stayed awake almost the whole day! He even got out of the chair and took a shower (his oxygen remained on). That's the first time he has done that in about two weeks. We played lots of Uno, Nintendo, and Guess Who today. He hasn't been pushing his morphine pump as much. Oxygen is still at 60 percent. He sang the alphabet song in his sleep during his nap this morning. I'm not sure what that was about, but he was telling Casey that's how you sing it right...

I did some schoolwork with Casey and Meghan today, and that felt good. Patrick and I left Grandma and Pockie in charge, and we escaped the hospital for two hours. Boy, was it ever good to see the outside world.

If there are people you haven't asked to pray for Logan, would you ask them? We need to get the whole world involved in this.

October 20, 1998: Greetings from Swedish Hospital. There are four crazy people playing Nintendo 64 at the same time. Seattle Sonics' game is holding Pockie, Patrick, Logan, and Gary mesmerized. Meghan and Casey are spending some time with Logan's Elvis CD.

Logan has had a pretty good day. I put a blanket and pillows on the floor. I got him down there, and we bounced a Super Ball back and forth. We also rolled cars to each other and played Sorry. He stayed on the floor for probably an hour and a half. It's nice to see him sit somewhere besides the chair. The physical therapist came up and had him do some stretches. They worked his arms and legs, and I think he enjoyed that.

His ANC dropped to 4,000 today. We'll see what it is tomorrow. Liver functions are quite elevated. I'm going to start him on a Shaklee product that is good for the liver. Kidney functions look fairly good. He had Tylenol three times again today. His highest fever was 102, but didn't last as long, thank God! He has felt pretty good, and his color is great. He looks healthier.

Doctors again cautioned us against false hope, but seemed encouraged. It's been eleven days since they told us they expected him to die. He's sixty days posttransplant, and his graft seems to be working well. Isn't that exciting? They did another chest x-ray today and said there is no change. Obviously, it's going to be a slow process, but as long as he is completely healed, we have all the time in the world. Thank you for your prayers. God bless you all.

October 21, 1998: Today is not a good day. Logan is fevering really bad. It started at 4:00 a.m. and won't let up. He's trying hard to fight it. Pockie is putting cold cloths on him and changing them often. It doesn't take long for his body to warm them up. His blood pressure is high, and his pulse is quite accelerated. The doctors came in this morning and said things don't look good. He is just not making any progress one way or the other. We are at a standstill. It has been almost two weeks since they first told us he has Aspergillus. Normally it would have already progressed to death. We are just here having our good days and our bad days. We see positive signs at times, and then we see other symptoms that don't change. It's frustrating. Extremely stressful.

The kids are going crazy. They have been cooped up for so long. They have been so good, but this is hard on them; it's hard on all of us. It's hard to watch such a brave, sweet child fight for his life day after day. I struggled, wondering, "Am I doing enough for Logan? Am I still being a good mom to Casey and Meghan? Are they going to look back and resent me?" Casey was being a bit naughty this morning, and Patrick yelled at him. I picked him up and held him but had to put him down when Logan had to pee. He resents the lack of attention, I think.

I pray that this fever is his last. When the fever is gone, so is his infection. Wouldn't that be wonderful? Wouldn't it be great if God just reached down His hand and said, "Okay, fungus, be gone!" Just like Jesus did with the lame man. "Pick up your mat and walk." Logan, get off your oxygen and walk out of this hospital; you are healed. That is my prayer.

October 22, 1998: It's Thursday evening, and we had a decent day today. Logan needed Tylenol two times today. He still ran fevers, but the highest was 102. He has felt pretty good. He's not as bright-eyed as he has been on his good days, but he's playing Uno right now. We played several games of bingo today. We also had a bubble-blowing session today. I gave him a glass of strawberry milk and a straw so he could blow bubbles to mix it all up. All three kids participated. They had a great time. Logan and Meghan carefully blew into the milk so the bubbles would come up but not go over the top.

Killing Leuk

Not Casey though! He blew his bubbles a little too hard, and we had a little spill. No biggie, though; he had fun. This is a great exercise for Logan's lungs. His CO_2 levels keep rising. This isn't a good thing. We are really pushing him to take deeper breaths and blow out harder.

Infectious-disease people came in today and said they are switching him to another form of amphotericin. This one will enable him to get a higher dose without as much toxicity. He can't get any more of the one he's on now. The nurse told me they don't think it will do any good because Logan is going to die anyway. I had a hard time with that. I let her know that she's not God, and she can't tell me what's going to happen with Logan. She said in all the years she has been here, she has only seen one or two survive Aspergillus. I told her Logan is not a statistic; he's Logan!

Talk about a blow! Why do they do this? We have our faith and belief that Logan will be healed. She can't take that away from us, but it can be depressing. We need to stay positive to help Logan through this. Hearing comments like that doesn't help.

Patrick and I called Logan's attending doctor in to talk to us after that. He still feels that Logan is at a plateau. No better/no worse. He says usually when someone stays the same, it is inevitable that they will take a turn for the worse. He has a better way of talking with us. After each bad thing he says, he tells us he hopes and prays it will be different. He sees the positives, not just the negatives. I'm not going to let it get me down. I will stay focused on our Lord. It is to him that I will look for answers. The doctors are just tools, not God.

Last night Patrick and I went out to dinner together. Then we picked Casey and Meghan up from the hospital and spent the night together in the apartment. That was what we all needed. We are much more refreshed today. Casey and Meghan even got along! They had fun playing together. For those of you who know them, you will understand that this was a miracle. They fight constantly. Mom and Dad were on duty last night.

They were up constantly with Logan, but they enjoy being his primary caretakers. They love him so much. Dad has to fly home today, but he'll be back in a few days.

Logan watched the videotape the church sent us today cheering him on. He had a big smile on his face when he realized how much he was loved. I don't think he can grasp the vastness of how deeply he is loved by so many. I tell him constantly how loved he is.

Please pray that this fungal infection will just go away! His belly is bigger. We thought it was going down, but it was actually just going lower and around the back. His ANC dropped to 3,700. They are starting him back on the GCSF shots tonight. Please continue to pray and remind others. Logan IS STILL HERE. The doctors did NOT expect him to be. It will be two weeks tomorrow since they told us. Let's pray we will show them that our God DOES do miracles.

October 23, 1998: I have a few praises to share. Logan has remained fever-free for the WHOLE DAY! Isn't this awesome? This evening it got up to ninety-nine, but they don't consider that a fever. Praise God! Also, they did his amphotericin earlier than normal. He got Demerol before it was administered and twice during it. The chills weren't as bad. It's over now, and he's watching a movie. Another praise is that his ANC is 7,200 today. Wow! We're happy about that.

The doctors told us this morning that his lungs don't sound as "wet" today. Also, his belly is a lot softer. Of course, we take these as positive signs. On another note, Logan slept almost the whole day. He's only really been awake for about an hour. He slept till four o'clock this afternoon and then was awake only a short period of time before he went back to sleep. He has complained of feeling worse during his short awake periods. He's complaining of a headache, being sore, and just not feeling good. I'm thinking that he's about over the hump. His fever is gone, and he just needs to work the last "yucky" things out of his body. I'm anticipating tomorrow will be an AWESOME DAY.

Killing Leuk

His liver functions were terribly high today. They have never been that high, and that's definitely a concern. Normally they test it every other day, but they will test again tomorrow to see what it is. Please pray it will be lower.

Casey is spending the night at the Jensens' house to play with Matt, who is seven. Meghan is spending the night in the apartment with Mom and my friend Dorothy, who just flew in. It's just Logan, our friend Gary, Patrick, and I tonight. I'm hoping Patrick will get some sleep tonight. He's up almost the whole night EVERY night. If Logan whispers, he jumps out of bed and goes running to him. He's such a wonderful and devoted father. Lucky for me that he is a night owl and that I do better early mornings. We balance each other out pretty darn well.

Thank you for your continued prayers. We love you all.

Thirteen

Saying Good-Bye Never Hurt So Bad

*H*ere is the final e-mail update I sent from the hospital before our world collapsed:

October 24, 1998: Last night was a good night. He is still fever-free. He woke up several times to go to the bathroom. This was without the diuretic. I think that's great. His pulse is down for the first time in a LONG time. Instead of beating 150 beats per minute, he's at 100. However, his breathing has worsened. He had to be turned up to 80 percent oxygen, and he's still struggling to breathe well on that. His head is still hurting, and he is coughing up a lot of blood. The doctors feel the Aspergillus has moved into his sinus passages, possibly his brain. They feel they infection is worsening.

How can there be so many positive things going on, like no fever, better heart rate, softer belly, at the same time as these other things? I asked Patrick how many ulcers we were going to have. He replied, "As many as it takes to get him through this." I agree, but I am stressed from the rocky road we are traveling. This morning I thought it was over. Now he's watching TV and doing fairly well. My hopes are high one moment, and I'm scared the next. When I look at him and see that he's not doing well, I don't know what *to think anymore. I am numb, yet I am still praying for a miracle. In one moment God can reach down and heal him. How we pray for this.*

• • •

After I wrote this last e-mail, Dorothy and I went for a walk outside. I told her that I really couldn't take much more. My baby was in so much pain, and I didn't want him to suffer anymore. But I just couldn't let my firstborn son go. How could I?

When we returned from our walk, I read Logan the last chapter of the Goosebumps book I had been reading to him, *The Boy Who Learned to Fly*. I knew the time was drawing near. Logan was weak, but he acknowledged his appreciation for the book. He loved it when we read to him. Patrick asked me, "Is he dying?" I replied, "I don't know." But I did know he was leaving us that night. I just couldn't say the words.

We sent word for Dad to come back. Ernie, Ginny, Gary, Dorothy, Casey, Meghan, Kevin, Erik, Waleen, and Larry were all at the hospital. There may have been more; we lost count. At one point Logan sat up, ripped off his oxygen mask, and said, "I want to go there, the door behind Ms. Dorothy." There was no door. I knew without a shadow of a doubt that Logan saw the door to heaven open. He took a big slug of Pepsi. The mom in me told him he shouldn't be drinking that. Really? What a dumb thing to say. I was still trying to pretend all was okay.

We sat there around Logan and rubbed his body and poured out our love on him. I stood up and said, "Logan, I am going to take out my contacts; I will be right back." I had no sooner turned my back when I heard Patrick cry out, "No!" and then he removed Logan's oxygen mask. I hit him and said, "Put it back on!" He said, "We lost our boy. He's gone!"

We all cried as we called for the nurse. She summoned the doctor and he pronounced him deceased at 10:10 on Saturday night, October 24, 1998. We said our good-byes to him and thanked him for being such a good son, grandson, and brother. The hospital allowed us to spend the night in the room with Logan. Casey slept next to his brother one last time. It was the most precious and loving act I had ever witnessed.

Later I sent one last e-mail: "Our precious baby died tonight. He's with Jesus now. God bless you all."

I think Logan chose to go in that moment because he knew two things: I had turned my back, and his beloved Pockie hadn't reached the hospital yet. He knew the two of us couldn't bear to watch him take his last breath. The little stinker always tried to make things easier for everyone.

The following days were a blur. I remember going back to the apartment and locking myself in the bathroom. I sat in the tub and just cried. I refused to eat, and I refused to talk to anyone on the phone. I just cried. Meghan and Casey were beyond distraught. They started sleeping with us. The four of us banded together and tried to comprehend what had just happened.

Mom and Dad took over. They made all the arrangements to have Logan's body shipped home and scheduled flights for us. Our church family took charge of his service and arranged everything.

I remember when Pastor Dennis came over. I couldn't even sit up and talk. I just laid my head on Patrick's lap and cried the whole time. I managed to give them enough information so they could have some special songs played. Pictures were there, a video was made, the programs were done—all by special church members. Thank goodness for that.

We held a private visitation for Logan at the funeral home. It was tough seeing him that last time. His face was so swollen. I put the quilt Granny made for him tightly around his face so he would look more like the Logan we knew. The next night we had a very large funeral for him. So many people from church, the community, friends, and even his pediatrician from Anchorage came. Logan was definitely honored.

Fourteen

Trying to Cope

Shortly after Logan died, I began to write. It was my way of expressing my hurt and anguish. *This is one of the pieces I wrote shortly after his death, on November 27, 1998*:

As children, we all had superheroes—those characters we admired and wished we could be. What exactly did these characters have that we wanted? Strength? Courage? The ability to make a difference in the world? The power to fight evil? As adults, we tend to forget about superheroes. We're too mature to think someone could be all that our beloved superheroes could be. As a parent, I found my true superhero: my son Logan. He had all that my superhero could have. He had the ultimate strength and courage. He made a difference in the lives of thousands. He showed me that God, through him, was fighting the evil called cancer.

Logan showed me how to be brave and how to face fears with dignity, grace, and strength. He showed me what it means to have unselfish love. He taught me to put others first. He showed me how to overlook my own needs and focus on others. He never put himself first. His needs weren't important to him. He needed to be there for those who needed him.

Killing Leuk

Logan went through twenty months of chemotherapy, radiation, and an umbilical cord transplant. He laughed through the vomiting and made jokes to cope with the pain. He went out of his way to make others feel good. He always had a twinkle in his eye and a smile on his face.

Logan truly cared about others. He cared about their pain. He waved to the children who would go by his hospital room. He always had a smile to give away. He didn't sit in bed crying, "Why me?" He made the best of his situation and enjoyed his time on earth.

My son is now an angel in heaven. You see, Jesus called him home on October 24, 1998. Eleven years and four months since our Heavenly Father loaned him to his father and me. We miss him so much, but we know we will see our "superhero" again.

Here I was at a crossroads. I had two small children to take care of and a husband who was also grieving. We went from a family of five to a family of four. Just like that. Life was different, and it was never going to be the same.

We tried so hard to focus on Meghan and Casey. We got them involved in sports, and we took them to counseling. We went as a family, and we also had them seen individually. I took them to grief-support groups for siblings. We tried to find ways for them to be involved in honoring their brother. Casey picked out a tree at Wonderland Park, and we paid for the city to place a marker there with Logan's name. That tree is a huge, proud spruce tree. It stands tall and honorable, just like Logan did. Our family got involved in the Light the Night Walk with the Leukemia & Lymphoma Society. We raised thousands and thousands of dollars for cancer research and patient support.

Patrick, Sharmin, Gary, and I walked a 26.1-mile marathon in San Diego in Logan's memory in 1999. It was the same marathon Logan wanted to do, so we did it for him. Believe me, he was our whole inspiration. We held hands as we crossed the finish line and shouted, "Logan!" Logan wanted to be a research scientist and find a cure for blood cancers. We did everything we could to keep his memory alive.

I threw myself into the community as an active volunteer. Any way I could keep my mind occupied was a good thing. I volunteered for many different organizations and helped cofound the Compassionate Friends group in Wasilla. Compassionate Friends is a group for bereaved parents. After some time, I quit going. It just seemed to make the pain worse, not better. We held multiple blood and marrow drives in memory of Logan. Every time someone donated blood or got on the bone marrow registry, I knew Logan would feel honored. One of Logan's dear friends, Caitlin Huckins, registered as soon as she was old enough. It wasn't long before she was told she was a match for someone. She saved a man's life by donating her stem cells to him. A man lived because Logan had a friend who honored his memory.

Through it all, I continued homeschooling Casey and Meghan along with my niece Michelle and my goddaughter, Delanie. We did the best we could as parents. I was always so sad but thought I was showing enough love for Casey and Meghan. One day, I pulled up to the hockey rink for Casey's hockey practice, and Meghan said, "I feel like you love Logan more than you do Casey and me."

Oh, the gut-wrenching pain I felt hearing those words. I said, "Meghan, I have four chambers of my heart. One is for Daddy, one is for Logan, one is for Casey, and one is for you. The chamber I had for Logan is missing, so now I have three. I hurt for that missing chamber, but I still have three chambers, which means I love you three just as much." I hope she understood that.

I continued writing as a coping mechanism. *I wrote this in 2001*:

Suffering the Loss of a Child

Posttraumatic stress syndrome and grieving the loss of a child. What do these two things have in common? Most people, when they hear the words "posttraumatic stress syndrome," automatically think of the sufferings of a war veteran. A soldier who has either been tortured, harmed in some way, or has witnessed the harm or suffering of others. A soldier who has posttraumatic stress syndrome might be faced with lifelong suffering. Vivid-image flashbacks might happen at any time, even when least expected.

Witnessing the death of a child can cause posttraumatic stress syndrome. Someone who has experienced the death of his or her child might have vivid-image flashbacks of the child being tortured or in pain. I am not referring to the torturing a soldier might go through, I am talking about the torture of treatment for cancer. I'm talking about the parents who have had to watch their child fight to survive massive injuries due to a car wreck, a fire, or an attack. I'm referring to those parents who have watched their children fight to stay alive, only to watch their child's body slowly fail even as he or she fights.

I am one of those parents. I have three children. Meghan is my youngest, and she is nine. Casey is my middle child, and he is eleven. Logan is my oldest. He would have been fourteen on June 24, 2001. On February 18, 1997, Logan was diagnosed with acute lymphocytic leukemia. He was nine years old, the same age as Meghan is now, and when he died, he was the same age as Casey is now.

Kelly Marre

We flew from our home in Alaska to Children's Hospital in Seattle, Washington. Logan endured twenty months of chemo, radiation, many doctor appointments, and finally a cord-blood transplant. I watched my son bravely endure many needles poking into him. He had many surgeries. He had many spinal taps, some of which the doctors insisted on doing when Logan was awake. There were two occasions when Logan had a bone marrow biopsy while awake. He had many more of those under sedation. We watched him struggle to be brave. Logan endured as much in a cancer ward as a soldier might have endured in a torture chamber. It was painful, frustrating, and confining. If his blood counts weren't at a certain level, he couldn't even leave his room. At times, he felt he was imprisoned and had no way to escape. He wanted to be home; he wanted to be a normal child again.

As I reflect on what happened to Logan, I am too numb to even write all that he endured. To speak the words makes me feel the pain as if it were yesterday. I can't let myself go there, or I may never return to reality. I think it would be easy to escape into a world where I didn't feel the mental anguish. I have witnessed the death of dozens of children. I have cried with parents after their children succumbed to death. I have gotten close to these children. I would often wave to them as I walked past their rooms. I have gone in their rooms and held their hands. I've walked by the next morning, and their rooms have been empty. Gone in the middle of the night. I suffer from the pain of losing my own child, but I've also suffered the loss of so many beautiful young friends. I have firsthand experience with the anguish of death.

How does one survive the posttraumatic stress of losing a child? There is no right or wrong way. I've been judged by my way of grieving, and I have seen others judged by their way of grieving. Some may think my way of grieving might not be healthy, or they may think someone else isn't grieving "appropriately." There are so many things I can teach you regarding helping someone go through the grieving process after losing a child.

Killing Leuk

I have had a lot of support from people since Logan became ill. Most of those people have continued to be a great support to me. I have heard things, though, that make me just want to gasp for air. Sometimes people just don't realize how their choice of words can make a grieving parent feel. At Logan's service, a close friend said to Patrick, "Aren't you glad your vasectomy didn't work, and you got Meghan? At least you still have two kids." Ouch. What a slap in the face. He meant well, but it was a painful thing for my husband to hear.

Logan died just before Halloween. Just a month later, people were preparing for Thanksgiving. I ran into a lady I was acquainted with, and she asked me if I were ready for the holidays. I told her the last thing we wanted to do was celebrate Thanksgiving and we had chosen to paint the inside of my parents' house instead. She reminded me that we still have two children to think about (as if I didn't know). It had been less than a month since his death and she implied that we weren't considering anyone else's feelings except our own. Then there was the friend who said, "At least you only have two children to get ready." Oh, that hurt.

There have been many times when I have had to leave a store because I started crying suddenly. Something might just trigger a flashback and the tears would come on heavily. It was over two years before I could go into a store without having a panic attack. I became very frightened of crowds. I was afraid to go into a store because I was terrified I would run into someone I knew and they would think, "There's Kelly; she is the one whose son Logan died." Maybe I didn't want to be clumped into that group. I have talked with other grieving parents who have said that they have similar feelings. For some reason, public places are frightening for us.

I spent twenty months fighting for my son's life. I spent twenty months spending every second searching for a cure, talking to doctors, and holding Logan's hand during treatment. I spent twenty months trying to keep my family together, trying to support my other two children at the same time. When Logan died, I felt like my purpose in life died too. After all that time, what was my purpose now? Nothing was the same.

I couldn't go back to the "old life" because that didn't exist anymore. To go on was betraying Logan. To ever smile or laugh would be unthinkable. I had to find a balance, but how?

It has been two years and seven months since Logan died. To this day, I still count out five plates for the table but only take four out of the cabinet. When we go into a restaurant and we are asked, "How many?" I reluctantly say four although inside, I am screaming, "FIVE!" When people ask me how many children I have, I always say three, but I pray they don't ask me how old they are. When they do, I always start with Meghan, the youngest, then my middle child, Casey, and then I say my oldest son Logan would have been…Then the questions start. Sometimes it's overwhelmingly painful. But then there are other times when I need to speak of Logan and his battle.

I appreciate the friends who tell me of memories they have of Logan. I appreciate those who tell me they admire him and remember him. I appreciate the little boy down the street remembering Logan when a song we played during his service is on the radio. Logan had a wonderful friend who helped me plan a memorial walk each year for the Leukemia & Lymphoma Society. To see this young man, give up his time and put forth so much effort to honor the memory of his friend Logan, touches my heart so very much.

I'm so grateful to those who remember Logan's birthday and the anniversary of his death. The cards I get, the prayers I feel, all help me to get through the dark times. We have chosen different ways to honor Logan. My mom and dad named their boat The Logan J. They had a plaque made for the boat slip, one that dedicated the boat and slip to Logan. Logan spent many hours playing there, and it was one of his very favorite places. We bought a memorial tree and plaque at our local playground. I recently bought a brick at our new memorial garden. None of these things take the pain away, but knowing that others see his name and remember Logan and the battle he fought helps us get through our days.

A grieving parent may be experiencing posttraumatic stress syndrome. If you know someone who has experienced the loss of a child, I urge you to tread softly and carefully. Give the parent a lot of love, not judgment. Just as the Vietnam War veteran will always remember, so will a grieving parent.

I wrote this the same year.

The Dos and Don'ts for Helping a Grieving Parent

1. Do not say, "Your child is in a better place." We know that; we don't need you to tell us that. Instead, validate our pain and let us know you understand we hurt.

2. Do not tell us what our child would want us to do, feel, or say. Our child wouldn't want to be forgotten, and I think our child would want us to grieve for him. Instead, be understanding when we are depressed. We are not going to "get over it."

3. Don't tell us to "be positive" or "look on the bright side." We are grieving our children who have died! Let us grieve! You can't force us to be positive. Let us come to you without feeling judged. We are not going to be positive and carefree all the time.

4. Understand that our grief overpowers us at times. While we know we should always treat others with respect, there might be times when we are moody and even angry. Don't take it personally. At that moment, we might be remembering something painful. It's okay to ask us if we are having a bad grief day. In our family, we would simply say, "I'm having a bad Logan day."

5. Understand that we might become withdrawn. Maybe we used to like to do a lot of things but prefer to stay around the house now. We are not the same people anymore. Please don't expect everything to be the same.

6. Please don't call us up and tell us your child has some of the same symptoms as our child did when he was diagnosed. Think about the horrible flashbacks that will cause us. While we care about your child's health, please don't call us and ask us if those symptoms are similar. Call your doctor instead.

7. Please don't ask us if we are going to have another baby. That makes us feel as if you think our child can be replaced. That is a personal and a private decision. If grieving parents do have another child after the loss of a child, do not assume they are "over their child's death."

8. If you have any pictures or movies of our children, please make copies and share them with us. We are sad because we won't be able to get new pictures of our child. If you share old pictures with us that we might not have seen before, it will fill us with joy.

9. It would be wonderful to receive a collection of memories you might have of our child. Maybe a scrapbook with some pictures and descriptions of activities you did with our child. Any memory is a good one.

10. Don't give up on us. It might take a long time before you can catch a glimpse of what we used to be like, or maybe you will never see that person again. Take time to get to know the "new us." Continue being there for us. If we were friends before, we'll continue being friends even through the tough times.

Fifteen

TIME DOES NOT HEAL ALL WOUNDS

On October 24, 2016, it was eighteen years since Logan had taken his last breath here on earth. I wish I could say that things got easier and less painful over the years, but they haven't. We miss Logan desperately, and our world isn't the same.

As they grew up, whenever our children would accomplish something, they silently honored their brother. Casey always asked for the number 24 jersey in honor of his brother. When I received volunteer awards, I always accepted the awards in honor of Logan. Patrick and I tried hard to be good parents to Casey and Meghan, but I know they felt cheated at times. They couldn't just be normal children. I only hope that despite the many mistakes I made as a parent, they truly know how much I love and respect them. I am sorry they had a mother who wasn't always "present" in the moment. I hope they know that despite my grief, I did not love them any less.

My grandfather Marvin suffered from Alzheimer's, and my parents moved him to Alaska to live with them shortly before Logan was diagnosed. Grandpa was out of it a lot, but he knew Logan was sick, and he cried for him. Grandpa and Granny had had a little boy named Dana. Dana had died from encephalitis when he was almost five. Grandpa never got over that. Before he had Alzheimer's, he would share his grief with me and tell me how much he believed he had caused his son to get sick. He thought that because he wasn't a good enough person and made mistakes, he was to blame for Dana's illness and death. Years after he professed this to me, I could really understand the guilt and blame myself. He also mourned the death of his grandson, Billy Dee. Billy Dee was my aunt Connie's firstborn son. He was run over by a big truck and killed.

After Logan's death, Grandpa would often spend the days with us. I had a picture of Logan on the windowsill. Grandpa would point to it every single day and say, "See that boy? That's Logan. He died."

I would gently say, "I know, Grandpa; he's my son." He would be surprised every time I said that.

On Logan's birthday that first year after his death, we released balloons to honor him. Grandpa had one lucid moment, and with clarity in his eyes, he said, "I will never forget him." The next moment Alzheimer's took back the clarity, but at that moment, he hurt for his great-grandson. I became very close to my grandpa. He died about a year after Logan did. I really went into a dark depression after that. I started seeing a counselor again and briefly went on antidepressants.

I think the turnaround for me was when I started working full time. I was always occupied and was too busy to show my grief. I'm

not saying the grief wasn't there, but I learned to compartmental-
ize it better—to stuff it down and leave it for a while. My mind
was fully occupied. I had two children in high school and was just
trying to survive raising teenagers. Trust me; it wasn't easy. Not
only did they have the normal teen things to deal with, but they
were also the surviving siblings. I know they missed their brother
so much. Each year Casey would share that he didn't want to be
older because Logan never got past eleven. It broke my heart to
hear that he didn't think he deserved to grow up.

The day my precious mother told me she had been diagnosed
with breast cancer about sent me over the edge. Oh, how I grieved!
But the woman rocked it. After a mastectomy and chemotherapy,
she beat it and is considered cured.

Our family was riddled with cancer. I was very close to my uncle
Terry, who died of pancreatic cancer. I was also close to a great
aunt who died of ovarian cancer. My mother lost her father to
non-Hodgkin's lymphoma when she was four. Her mother died
of brain cancer when Mom was eighteen, and her sister, my aunt
Judy, died of breast cancer when she was in her early forties. So
many losses. Our family seems cursed with malignancy.

• • •

Before I knew it, my children were grown. They both married
their high school sweethearts. Meghan and her husband started a family right away and gave us a beautiful little granddaughter
named Olivienne. Things were going great, and we finally started
feeling some relief from our loss from the pain of losing Logan.
Olivienne didn't replace Logan, but she helped us find someone

else to love. And boy, did we love her! She was so sweet and funny. She reminded me of Logan. She talked at a very early age and we told her all about her Uncle Logan. She would point at his pictures and say, "Logan!"

In 2005, I started working with victims of domestic violence and sexual assault as a crisis intervention coordinator. In 2008, I accepted a position in probation. I had always wanted to be an FBI agent or a detective, and this was as close as I was going to get. I used to read the Trixie Belden, Nancy Drew, Hardy Boys, and Three Investigators series. I can't say I solved mysteries, but I was astute at identifying a lie anyway. I embraced the job and looked forward to going to work every day. I was finally feeling like I had begun to heal. I felt I had a purpose and that by helping others I could give back to society. I respected the offenders I worked with and grieved their poor choices. I preferred using counseling and teaching techniques over arresting when possible.

Sixteen

DIRTY NEEDLES AND SIDE EFFECTS

On July 23, 2014, I was out in the field doing an unannounced field visit on a prisoner my partner and I supervised. We worked for the State of Alaska, Department of Corrections, as probation officers. We supervised felons and misdemeanants on house arrest. One day, we decided to check on one man we suspected might be up to no good. We had gotten anonymous tips that drugs were being used in the home.

My partner, Mindy, stayed with the prisoner while I searched the residence. It didn't take long before I found used syringes. Our suspicions were correct; he had been cohabitating with a known drug user. I had the package of needles in my hand when I picked up something else. I accidentally banged the needles against my leg, and a used needle jammed into my leg so deeply I oozed blood. Being the professional I was, I didn't say anything to my partner until we had the guy secured in our transport vehicle and were on our way to the jail. I was a basket case, but I was on autopilot.

As soon as he was dropped off and the paperwork was finished, I made my way to the emergency room at our local hospital. I was assigned a doctor who portrayed himself as completely disinterested in me as a person or as a law enforcement officer. He stated the facts coldly and emotionlessly, telling me I was at risk for contracting HIV or hepatitis C. He told me I had to start on medication immediately. He didn't stay long enough to give me any information about how the medicine would affect me. Patrick was out of town, and I didn't want to ask anyone to come. I texted my mom. She offered to come sit with me. I said, "No Mom. If you show up, I will start crying. How would that look if a PO in full uniform started crying? I have to be strong." I really wanted my mommy, though.

The first thing I did after leaving the emergency room, was drive up to Meghan and Kirk's house and confess to them what had happened. As I sobbed, I told them I would understand if they didn't want me around Ollie until we knew if I had contracted a communicable disease. I would never do anything to harm our granddaughter. Meghan and Kirk wrapped their arms around me and assured me they were not concerned and felt their baby would be safe. The intensity of the relief I felt was almost tangible. I was relieved; I could continue being Grammie.

The first week that I took the medicine, I felt fine. I continued all my activities and smugly decided I was going to escape any side effects the pharmacist had warned me about. He had told me the biggest side effect was nausea. I hated throwing up, so I sure didn't want that! Soon I no longer wanted the decaf skinny lattes that I always got on Tuesdays and Fridays. The thought of them made me nauseous. Food started tasting funny, and nothing sounded good—not even my sugar-free chocolates! I felt extremely nauseous and out of breath.

Killing Leuk

I was in good shape; I could outwalk most people and did a lot of hiking, Zumba, and other exercise classes at our local gym. Soon, I gasped for air just carrying my gear bag to my car after work. I called my family doctor a few times, but each time his medical assistant told me I didn't have a choice: I had to stay on the medication.

Thirty days later I was finished with the medication, but the symptoms just got worse. One day I was driving home, praying that God would take the symptoms away and prevent me from getting HIV or Hep C. I remember pleading with God to spare me from that. I said, "God, there is no dignity in saying I have HIV or Hep C. I will be stigmatized. It's not like someone who gets a cancer diagnosis. Logan was perceived as honorable throughout his cancer diagnosis."

Suddenly, I felt with the upmost certainty that my fate had been changed forever on July 23, 2014, and my life would never be the same. It was the same feeling I had had on February 12, 1997, when I heard God say, "Will you still believe in me and share my love with others if your whole life is changed?" I was afraid. For some reason, God speaks to me in ways that are clearly meant to get my attention. I didn't say anything to Patrick or my family, but I knew I likely had leukemia.

I confided to my friend Kris that I was worried I had leukemia. Seventeen years prior, on February 17, 1997, our oldest son Logan had been diagnosed with leukemia. He was short of breath and had no energy. I will never forget the day when he told me he felt so weak. I was starting to understand how he felt. But aside from talking to Kris, I kept my worries to myself; I didn't want to sound paranoid. I made an appointment to see my doctor after my vacation.

Patrick was going on a business trip to Seattle, and I had decided to meet him there after his meeting. We knew we didn't want to stay in Seattle and tried to agree on where to go. I had always wanted to go to Idaho and talked him into going on an unplanned road trip. What I didn't tell Patrick before we left was that I suspected I had leukemia. Before we left, we went to our cabin on the Kenai Peninsula. Our cabin is our favorite place on earth because we love the solitude we have there. We had so much fun working together, with the help of family and friends, to build our oasis. I wasn't feeling well at all but wanted to help stack wood. I had no energy, and it was all I could do to carry a stick of wood. I was concerned but laughed it off while knowing deep inside that there was a serious problem.

Seventeen

CAREFREE ADVENTURE TURNS SERIOUS

The first night we drove to Newport, Washington, to see our friend Jim. Jim had been trying to talk us into visiting him for years. We were happy to finally accept his invitation. Jim had come up to Alaska in 1997 and had been part of Logan's adventure riding a dogsled for the Iditarod. He took a fantastic picture that we proudly display on our wall.

We had a pleasant evening with Jim and went out to dinner with his family and friends. I was feeling fairly well and put my concerns about my health to rest for the night. When we got back to his house, I decided to call it a night. I left the two men upstairs to catch up and climbed into bed feeling exhausted. The next morning, I woke up with a sore throat. The timing was terrible! We only had a few days of vacation, and I refused to let a sore throat ruin our trip. Besides having a sore throat, I was feeling achy and tired. I asked Patrick to go upstairs and mix me up some salt water to gargle. He came down with a cup of salt mixed with a teeny bit of water. Yuck. I went upstairs to make another cup of salt water, and by the time I got up there, I could hardly breathe. I could tell that Jim and Patrick were concerned, but I told them I was just overly tired. Patrick and I gathered our belongings and set out for our adventure in Idaho.

The only hotel I had reservations for was for our first night in a small town called Post Falls. I had Googled information about Post Falls before we left. The only attraction I had discovered was that the town boasted of having a buck knife Factory. That sounded fun, and we wanted to check it out. Post Falls is close to Coeur d'Alene, which was a place I had heard about and wanted to visit. Jim had suggested we start in Sand Point, Idaho, and then drive to Post Falls. Having been raised in a small town in Indiana, I appreciated the hometown feeling of Sand Point. There were so many beautiful old buildings, and I was eager to walk around the town. We started walking, but it wasn't long before we had to slow our pace down. I was having trouble catching my breath and was frequently stopping to sit. At one point I even sat down in a store we were in. I knew this wasn't good; something was very wrong with me.

A few weeks before we had left, Patrick and I had gotten blood tests done at our local health fair. We hadn't received the results before leaving Alaska. I knew I needed to see my labs. I texted our daughter-in-law, Kelsey, who was in her last year of nursing school. I asked her if she could check our mail to see if the hospital had mailed our results. The results were there, and she took a picture of the labs and told me what I already knew: "You need to see a doctor," she said. I immediately sent the results to my mother, and she called my doctor, David Barnes, who is a family friend. David told her I needed to find the closest emergency room and get a blood transfusion.

Killing Leuk

At that point I knew I needed to tell Patrick my suspicions about what was wrong with me. I wanted to prepare him. As we stood on the sidewalk in Sand Point, I put my hand on his chest and said, "Honey, there is something you need to know. I want you prepared for the worst. I think I have leukemia or lymphoma." Although the breathing issues were like Logan's, my other symptoms were like the ones my friend Kelly had when she was diagnosed with lymphoma. My chest felt like an elephant was sitting on it.

Of course, Patrick reassured me that I was just having residual effects from the medicine, and it was nothing serious. We agreed to check into our hotel, have lunch, and then go to the ER. I called my insurance company to see if there was a preferred hospital I had to go to. They told me any hospital was okay. I looked up hospitals and found one in Coeur d'Alene. I couldn't tell how big it was, and I sure didn't know whether it was a good hospital or not.

We had a delicious lunch and then asked our waitress how to find the hospital. She gave us three different routes to take. Listening to her change her mind on how to get there stressed me out more, and I found it even more difficult to breathe. I wondered if I just had some anxiety issue. We finally made it, and I signed in. The first thing I told the triage nurse was that I had recently been on prophylactic medication and showed her my blood test results. She weighed me, and I realized I had lost a few pounds in just a couple of weeks. After I was back in a room, they took some more blood from me. I again went through my story of being on the meds and asked the medical staff if they thought it was related. The ER doctor did some research and found that one of the medicines suppressed the bone marrow. When the results for the blood tests came back, we discovered I was even more anemic than I had been two weeks prior. The doctor told me I needed a blood transfusion right away and that we needed to figure out where I was bleeding from.

Since I was going to be admitted, I sent Patrick back to our hotel for clothes, makeup, and hair supplies. While he was gone, I took the opportunity to ask the doctor if he thought I had leukemia. He looked surprised and asked me why I thought that. I told him about Logan and how some of our symptoms were similar. He said, "I don't think you have leukemia because your white blood count is normal and so are your platelets. I think you may have an ulcer that is causing you to be anemic." Although an ulcer didn't sound fun, I preferred that over leukemia! I felt a little more confident that I was going to be okay. I figured I would just walk to my room, but they wheeled the whole bed to my new room. I was thinking, "Wow, this is a little overkill—I could have walked!" What I didn't know was that they put me on One North wing, which I later discovered was where the cancer patients go.

At this point I was confident everything would be okay. A new doctor came in and told me he needed to figure out where I was losing blood from and that they would transfuse me. He mentioned doing either an endoscopy or a colonoscopy. I told him I would take the first option. I figured I would be in and out within a matter of a day or two. After all, I could always follow up with my doctor at home. I sent Patrick back to the hotel to get some sleep. I was confident we would be able to continue our vacation. The next morning the same doctor came in and asked me about Logan. I was surprised he had heard the story I had shared with the ER doctor. I gave him an abbreviated version of our twenty months of Logan's brave battle with acute lymphocytic leukemia.

Killing Leuk

He listened carefully and then said, "I am sorry to tell you this, but we think you have leukemia too." I looked over at Patrick and saw the fear on his face. I knew then my response at that moment and attitude in the future had to be confident, positive, and encouraging to him and others. I calmly asked, "Okay, what steps do we need to take?" I looked at Patrick and said, "It's going to be okay." He burst into tears and hugged me tightly. I felt such love for this man who hurt so badly.

The pain of watching Logan struggle came rushing back. My greatest concern was about the pain my family would experience watching me go through similar treatment as Logan did. I didn't think they could take anymore. It had been sixteen years that month since Logan had died after contracting a fungal infection following an unrelated umbilical-cord stem-cell transplant. How could we go through this again? The anguish from losing Logan is as raw and painful today as it was then. February 17, 1997, was the second worst day of my life. Logan wasn't getting over his "virus"; he was tired, weak, and bruised. He had these funny little spots we later learned were called "petechiae." I didn't have petechiae, but I did have the shortness of breath and the exhaustion. This was an unwanted flashback of the past—a flashback to terrible memories of how sick our boy had been.

Now, seventeen years later, it was my turn to be told, "You need a bone marrow biopsy to determine if you have leukemia." I guess the doctor thought it would somehow ease the emotional pain if he told us he thought I had a different type of leukemia than Logan had and that it wasn't genetic. Maybe it did help. I certainly didn't want to think Logan had gotten sick because I carried some defective gene and he got the disease before me.

The biopsy was done right in my room, and the doctor made Patrick leave. He said, "I don't need two patients." I didn't want to go through that without him, but I put on a brave front and braced myself. I was no stranger to bone marrow biopsies; Logan had had dozens. Two were done while he was awake, and after that I said, "Never again." It doesn't matter how much they numb you; it is uncomfortable! I was determined to be stoic and silent. But at one point, I said, "Shit, that hurts! It feels like you are using a drill on my hips!" The doctor said, "Well, actually I kind of am!" I then apologized for cussing. He said, "You handled this so much better than the marines I have done this on!"

A short time later, Dr. Mulvey let us know the preliminary report was back and confirmed what we already knew: I had leukemia-specifically an aggressive type of leukemia called, "Acute Myelogenous Leukemia". I immediately felt at peace and said, "I have a win-win situation. If I die, I can go to heaven and be with Logan. If I beat this thing, then I can stay here with my family and be a grandma to all those grandchildren I hope to have."

Eighteen

BREAKING THE NEWS AND STARTING CHEMO

I picked up the phone and broke the news to family one by one. I had to be strong because if I fell apart, so would everyone else. No matter how much I tried to prepare myself before going to the hospital, my head was still spinning with the reality of my diagnosis. A million things were going through my head, but foremost was "What do I need to do to kill this thing?" I never once thought about not doing everything I could do to survive.

Later, when things calmed down, I was shocked to realize how badly I wanted to live. When Logan died, Patrick and I had both said we wouldn't do treatment if we had cancer because we had no faith in the medical system. Sixteen years after his death, I was ready to slay the monster inside of me. The guilt crept in as I asked myself why I deserved to live when Logan didn't. It didn't seem right that I was fighting so hard. The feelings of failing him came rushing back.

Dr. Mulvey asked us where we wanted to do treatment. Patrick and I looked helplessly at one another. We certainly wanted the best care with the best treatment possible for survival. Could we get that in Alaska? We sure couldn't with Logan—we had lived in Seattle most of the twenty months of his battle. But could we really be uprooted again? Dr. Mulvey made it somewhat easy for us; he called the hospitals in Alaska and was told no one could treat my rare type of AML up there. But now what? We absolutely did not want to go back to the city where Logan had died. Seattle hadn't killed Logan, but the thought of the city brought out bitter feelings. Could we really deal with all those emotions again?

For years, we had hated hospitals. We couldn't step foot in one without feeling the grief hit us like a ton of bricks. Patrick would make every excuse he could not to go. I would put on a brave front, but felt like I was dying inside every time I went to visit someone. In Coeur d'Alene, we realized for the first time in years that we were in a hospital and feeling somewhat comfortable. We were impressed with the nurses, and everyone seemed to genuinely care about us. Dr. Mulvey told us Kootenai Hospital, the one we were in, was affiliated with the Mayo Clinic and had a study if we were interested. I looked at Patrick, and he nodded affirmatively. We would stay in Coeur d'Alene. We were going to be so far away from everyone we knew. Anticipated loneliness set in.

That night there was a knock at the door. Patrick opened it, and I heard a familiar voice. One of Logan's greatest supporters was our friend Gary. Gary lived in Renton, Washington, when Logan was sick. He had come to the hospital every single day. The support he so freely gave helped us through the worst time of our lives. There stood our faithful friend once again. He had driven six hours from his new home in Arlington, Washington. He rushed over to my bed with tears in his eyes and gave me a big, reassuring hug. We were no longer alone.

It wasn't long before word about my diagnosis spread like wildfire. So many wanted to help in any way they could. We had plans that first night in Idaho to have dinner with Jan, our former Alaskan neighbor. I called to tell her the news, and she graciously offered any help she could give and invited our friends and family to stay with her while visiting us. It was comforting to know she was in Coeur d'Alene.

Our biggest dilemma was finding an affordable place to live. We put our daughter in charge of researching that. One day she was busy calling about places when a family friend phoned her. Meghan said, "I can't talk right now, I'm trying to find my parents a place to live." Our friend Tammy said, "That's why I'm calling you! My sister has a home in Coeur d'Alene, and she wants them to stay there!"

We were showered with blessings each day. Family and friends made plans to come, and soon they made sure we had everything we needed. Both of us had the full support of our employers. Patrick had worked for E. J. Bartells for almost twenty-five years. When Logan was sick, his company had been a tremendous support and helped us so much. There were two new owners, Rick Smith and Brian Farnsworth. Both were just as supportive as the former owners. They immediately told Patrick that they would help any way they could and he wasn't to worry about work. They insisted he focus on me. My coworkers immediately offered me leave so I could continue getting paid and have insurance. We were overwhelmed with gratitude and thankfulness. We had an army standing beside us ready to go into battle and fight. We were never going to be alone.

I spent Friday and Saturday night in the hospital and was released on Sunday. I have no recollection of leaving the hospital. I'm not sure if my brain decided it just couldn't think anymore, or if I was so emotionally stunned that my brain was shutting down. All I remember is being at the hotel and waiting to hear from Dr. Mulvey. We had decided to participate in the study. After all, one more drug working to kill this "thing" was good, right? We got the call we had been waiting for. Dr. Mulvey told me I had been accepted into the study. I cheered and said, "That's so awesome!" There was a brief silence, and he drily replied, "I'm glad you are so excited. Now get your butt down here now!"

We drove to the cancer clinic in Post Falls. It was a surreal experience knowing I was the patient and this wasn't going to just go away. We were pleasantly greeted and given a bunch of paperwork to fill out. They put us in a room to speak to us privately. The nurse explained the process and brought in the study nurse to tell us about the pills I would be taking on the study. She explained that I would have five rounds of chemo and that the pills were to be taken the first three days of each round. I was starting the induction phase that day.

The nurse put a ham sandwich in front of me and said, "You need to eat this or you will get sick." I groaned at the thought of being sick, but I sure didn't feel like eating. I took one bite, and my appetite returned! I gobbled the sandwich up, much to the delight of Patrick and Gary who had been trying to coax me into eating for days! She then handed me the pills. I was to take six pills twice a day for three days. They had to be taken twelve hours apart and always with food. Chemotherapy had officially begun.

The first day wasn't too bad. I was tired and a little bit nauseous, but overall I was doing okay. On day two I had noted down how I was feeling: "Day 2 of chemo pills—I don't feel so well. I'm thankful Patrick and Gary are here to take care of me, and I can't wait for Mom, Meghan, and Olivienne to come." On day three, I wrote, "I woke up at 0500 sicker than a dog. Yuck. I'm trying not to wake anyone. Mom, Meghan, and Olivienne arrived, and I am so blessed. I'm praying for a good day on Meghan's twenty-third birthday. God, please give me energy and a day without nausea. I want her to have a good day. I want Olivienne to be comfortable around me and not afraid."

That afternoon I insisted we get out of the house and do something fun. We made it as good of a day as we could by celebrating the birth of our youngest child. We were just thankful to be together. On day four it was time to be admitted. Boy, did I dread going back to the hospital. I dreaded IV chemo and being confined to a room. I kept thinking I would wake up from the bad dream and be back in Alaska.

When I got up that morning, I was violently ill. I was on my knees in front of the toilet retching and feeling like my insides were going to come out of my mouth. I started to laugh at a memory that came rushing back. We were in Swedish Hospital, and Logan wanted to take a bath. I was running his water, and he was kneeling in the same position I currently was, vomiting repeatedly. I had felt helpless knowing there was nothing I could do to stop his pain and discomfort. Suddenly, he had stood up, wiped his mouth, and said, "Is there anything else that needs fixin', ma'am?" I looked at him strangely and said, "What on earth are you talking about?" He had responded, "I'm the naked plumber, ma'am, and I'm here to help." At that moment, I knew whatever I was going to go through was nothing compared to what Logan went through. I stood up and resolved to be brave and strong like Logan.

By the time we got to the hospital, my resolve was shaken a bit. I was so sick, and they told me I needed pain medication before they put my Hickman line in. I have adverse reactions to pain medication. Three things may happen: I throw up, I hallucinate, or I have nightmares. I can handle hallucinations and nightmares, but remember, I hate throwing up! We finally agreed on a medication, and they wheeled me into the procedure room. I was awake when they put in a catheter that went from my neck to my heart. The technicians were joking with me and asked me all kinds of questions about Alaska. I soon became known as the "Alaska Girl."

After my line was in, I was wheeled to the room that would become my new temporary home. I was a little nervous about having the Hickman. After one of Logan's many procedures, a technician had somehow grabbed his line and snapped one of the lumens clean off! Logan was so mad. He kept saying, "You broke my line! You broke my line!" I decided to guard mine with my life.

It was time for the IV chemo to begin. They hooked me up to a triple IV pole that allowed for multiple medications and fluids to be given at the same time. I named it Tad because if the pole was going to be hanging out with me for an indeterminate amount of time, it was going to have a name! "Tad Pole" seemed an amusing name for such an annoying piece of equipment. Tad followed me everywhere! I couldn't even go to the bathroom alone. It was worse than having little toddlers around. Instead of hearing "Mommy, mommy, mommy," I was hearing "beep, beep, beep." I would make him stop temporarily by pushing the silent button, but what I really wanted to do was shoot him with my Glock. However, as annoying as Tad was, he was giving me medication that would hopefully save my life.

One of the drugs was given slowly over a period of twenty minutes. The nurse had to sit beside my bed and manually push it into my Hickman line. I was very nervous and decided to listen to the praise and worship CD my friend Laura had made for me. I put the CD in, closed my eyes, and immersed myself in the music. I felt God's presence as I visualized the medication attacking the cancer cells. I was filled with a feeling of peace.

Soon my room was filled with friends and family. The nurses had to round up extra chairs to hold all my guests! They were shocked to hear most of the people there had flown from Alaska just to be with me. My friend Pam flew in from California and showered me with gifts. I looked around the room and realized how loved I was. Each visit was a blessing from God. We spent time laughing and rejoicing for the time we had together. Underneath the laughter, I sensed the worry and concern my loved ones had for me. It was especially hard on my son and daughter. Although they were very young when Logan was sick, they hadn't forgotten how difficult it was. I could see they were reliving that experience. I saw the fear in their eyes as they wondered if their mom was going to die too.

We were anxiously awaiting the results of three marker tests. The marker tests would define what subtype of leukemia I had so the doctors could properly treat me. If the markers came back "good," it meant I had a better chance to survive. Dr. Mulvey reassured me that having a "rare" type of AML didn't mean my chance of recovery was necessarily compromised. What mattered most were the results of the markers. The test results slowly came in. The first two tests came back in my favor. We were ecstatic and celebrating! It seemed to take forever for the last test to come back. My nurse practitioner gave me the news: it was negative! I called my family and announced the results on Facebook. We were on top of the world. Leuk had no hold over me, and I was going to kick his butt to kingdom come.

Dr. Mulvey came in that night, and I told him we were celebrating the results of the last test. He looked at me compassionately and said, "Kelly, we wanted this particular test to be positive." I was crushed. I tried to act as though everything was okay, but he had learned to read my emotions by then. He told me to stop worrying—that last test was the least important of all of them. I held back the tears. How would my family and friends cope with this setback?

Nineteen

PLAN A ALL THE WAY

From the beginning, I was determined to be on "Plan A." Plan A was five rounds of chemo with no complications, and then I would go home and resume my normal life. But the news about the last marker stopped me cold. I decided I could either live in fear or trust in the Lord. I chose to trust Him. I was filled with peace again and resolved to fight even harder. Every day I would put a mask on, grab Tad, and go for a walk around One North. Usually Mom or Patrick went with me. On the days when I had lots of company, we would all go! What a scene to behold—all those people walking down the hall pushing Tad. As fun as that was, there was a cloud hanging over our heads. The anniversary of Logan's death was coming up, and I was in the hospital. Sixteen years before, we had watched our son take his last breath in a hospital. The pain was just too much to bear. We hurt, and we were scared.

It was just after midnight, so technically it was October 24, the anniversary of Logan's death. I was alone and wide awake reliving that last night with him. I called for the nurse to bring me

Ativan. Ativan was helpful for nausea, anxiety, and sleep. My nurse, Kristina, came in with the pills and asked me what was wrong. I burst into tears and told her it was the anniversary of Logan's death. We spent well over an hour talking about him. She hugged me with tears streaming down her face. She wiped them away in disbelief and said, "I never cry! What is going on? Maybe I should rethink being an oncology nurse." I laughed and told her that she was a human with compassion and it was okay to show it.

It was a sleepless night despite the medicine. In the morning, every nurse, physician's assistant (PA), and doctor who walked into my room acknowledged our loss and showed us compassion. It affirmed we were being treated in the right place. The hospital may not have been large, but we were getting excellent care from a caring staff.

We were determined to honor Logan on this day. The best way we could do that was for me to try as hard as I could to beat this thing. Thankfully I had an entourage to encourage me. Mom, Dad, Gary, my cousin Holly, and my friend Pam took Tad on a walk. Patrick didn't feel like walking so he stayed in the room. Pam, Holly, and I had something special planned to help our troubled mood. We had the song "I'm an Overcomer" by Mandisa cued up and ready to go. Pam hit the play button, and she, Holly, and I started dancing in the hallway. The looks on Gary's and my parents' faces were hysterical. They were shocked. We got lots of stares, but we didn't care.

We danced like it was 1999 as we cheered that I *was* an overcomer and with God's help, would beat this monster inside of me. We danced back to the room to "Eye of a Tiger." Later, we went outside and made a video of our "I'm an Overcomer" dance. We realized we couldn't quit our day jobs to become dancers, but we had the time of our lives. We were filled with joy. We honored Logan.

I spent my sleepless nights plotting how to prank my nurses. I don't know what came over me, as normally I am a nice and serious person! I thought about some of the jokes Logan had played on his nurses and doctors. I came up with my own evil plans. At the beginning of my IV chemo, my nurse, Charles, had me print and sign my name each night to make sure my cognitive abilities hadn't been compromised. The second night, I wrote a different name in different handwriting. I handed it back to Charles and waited for him to notice. His eyes got real big, and he looked at me fearfully thinking I had lost it. I laughed and said, "Got you!"

Another night I hid in the bathroom with a blanket over my head and a duck call in my mouth. When I heard Charles come in, I jumped out of the bathroom and blew that duck call. I doubled over laughing as he jumped and yelled. He told me he would be right back after he changed his pants. Logan would have been proud.

Just when things seemed to be going well, I developed a strange rash on my back and weird spots on my breasts. Dr. Mulvey declared it to be shingles. All nurses had to wear protective gowns and masks when they came into my room. They didn't want to expose other patients. I was told I could still go on my multiple walks per day, but I had to change into a fresh gown and robe each time. That was a pain, but worth the effort. There was no way I could lie in that bed twenty-four hours a day. They would have to transfer me to the psych ward because I would totally lose it!

They called in a specialist named Dr. Souvenir. Yes, Mom and I giggled like schoolgirls every time we said his name. Dr. Souvenir announced that I didn't have shingles; I was having a reaction to my Hickman, and it had to come out. It was a frustrating few days because each doctor and nurse who looked at my rash had a different opinion. The Hickman was to come out immediately; no; let's wait and see; get it out now; maybe it's looking better...oh, she has a fever; let's get it out. Finally, it was out, and a PICC line was put in. My strange heart palpitations stopped.

Before long, the day I had been dreading arrived. I was washing my hair on day fourteen, and a huge clump of hair fell out. I laughed and said, "So it has begun." I put my pretty highlighted hair on a paper towel and showed all my visitors. I took this surprisingly well! The same thing happened the next day. My hair was so tangled I had to have my certified nursing assistant (CNA) comb through it. I didn't understand why it was tangled, and she explained the hair falling out was wrapped around my rooted hair, thus tangling them together.

When my niece Michelle arrived that morning, I asked her to cut my hair short. She had never cut hair before and was a little nervous. She gave me an adorable cut, which I proudly displayed to all my nursing staff and friends. I was hoping to wear that cute style for a while. However, the next morning another huge amount of hair fell out. Again, the tangles were so bad I couldn't comb it myself.

Killing Leuk

I'd had enough; it was time to shave it. Mom went to buy clippers, and I tried to build up courage. I appointed Patrick to do the honors. I felt sorry for him because I knew it was hard on him. He started cutting and clipping. I sat there without saying a word. The tears were streaming down my face, and I was angry for being so upset over my hair. I wanted to be brave like Logan was. When his hair had started falling out, we had celebrated by having a shaving party. Casey had shaved his head to show support for his brother. Patrick had offered to shave his head to support me. It was a sweet gesture, but I liked his hair too much.

I tried putting on a brave front as I put on the hat Patrick had bought me. I announced I was tired and silently cried myself to sleep. A few hours later, my nurse Valerie woke me up. She was a sweet, tiny thing who was normally very quiet. She stood beside my bed and said in her best stern voice, "You are getting out of this bed and going for a walk with me!" I did as she commanded and walked out of my room for the first time with no hair.

My brother and his wife arrived the next day. I had been so excited to see them, but I was self-conscious and nervous about their reaction. Mark and Sharmin flew into the room, hugged me, and declared that I had the most perfectly shaped head ever and could totally pull off being bald! They could only spend a few days and were determined to encourage us and take our minds off things. We spent the afternoon playing cards and reminiscing about family events. On Halloween, they took off and went to the store to find me something to wear. They came back with a huge bag of goodies and proceeded to dress me up like I was some mannequin who needed to come to life. It was hilarious to watch them as they pulled one thing after another out of the bag. They would put something on me and then grab the camera. "Quick, take her picture! Okay, now put this on her!" Finally, they deemed me appropriately dressed for our walk. I walked out with a pink cowboy hat, huge glasses, fake beard, and my mask. We were going dancing with Tad. My nurse Andrew saw me and jumped. I certainly surprised him!

Twenty

JAILBREAK!

November 1, the day I had been waiting for, had finally arrived. I was being released from jail. I mean hospital. I could go back to our rental home in Coeur d'Alene. No more being woken up several times to have my temperature taken and no more having my urine measured each day! I could pee and not have to show it to anyone! I was free to do whatever I wanted, or so I thought...

My mother and husband watched me like hawks. "It's time to take your temperature, it's time for your nap, it's time for your medicine, it's time to eat." I gave up arguing. I did as I was told and thanked God for my caregivers. When I wanted to go on a walk, one of them always went with me. I was extremely loved and cared for. Soon they both needed to go home and take care of things. My friend Darlene came to stay with me. Darlene is a nurse, so they knew they were leaving me in good hands. Darlene took her orders from Mom seriously. She cleaned per the schedule Mom had instructed and made sure I ate and took my medicine. She had brought me lots of gifts, including a biker-chick leather hat. She was as eager to dress me up as Mark and Sharmin had been.

My days revolved around my clinic appointments, blood tests, and transfusions. I alternated between needing red blood cells and platelets. This was my new life. How I longed to be home and back at work. I tried to keep my spirits up, but I felt worthless. I didn't even have the energy to cook a meal for my husband. I no longer had my independence. One thing I wouldn't give up was my walks. No matter how low my hemoglobin got or how hard it was to breathe, I would put on my coat and go for a walk. I wasn't going to give up fighting, and I needed to rebuild my strength and stamina.

I wanted to go home for a visit so badly. My medical team would not allow it until my counts came up to a safe level for me to fly. I was neutropenic, meaning I had no immune system to fight off germs. On November 14, my counts were finally at the level they needed to be. My bone marrow biopsy was scheduled for the next day. Meghan and Patrick drove me to the clinic, and Meg and I went back to the infusion room. They put us in a private room with a bed and started handing me pills to ease the discomfort. My PA, Megan, came in and numbed me by inserting a large needle filled with medication into my hip. She allowed Meghan to stay in the room after we reassured her she would be able to handle watching the procedure. Meghan was a great support. She held my hand and said, "Mom, I want you to breathe like I did when I was having Ollie." I chuckled at the role reversal. She became Mom, and I did as she instructed. Soon it was over, and we left hoping the results would come back showing I was in remission.

Killing Leuk

If I was in remission, I could go home for a week. Otherwise, I would be back in the hospital getting chemo, and plans would be made for a bone marrow transplant. Mom, Dad, and Casey came in the next day, and Kirk came the following day. Kelsey was unable to come, as she was busy with nursing school. Since we didn't know if I was going to be able to go home, we planned to celebrate Thanksgiving in Idaho. Mom and Meghan made a delicious dinner, and we celebrated being together. I couldn't help but wonder if this would be my last Thanksgiving. No one said anything, but I knew they were thinking the same thing.

On the seventeenth the kids left, and it was just Mom, Dad, Patrick, and I. The house seemed so quiet. No more noise from the pitter-patter of our grandbaby's feet. The next day we had an appointment at the clinic. We were hoping the results of the bone marrow biopsy would be in. The examination rooms were small, so usually just one person would go back with me. Patrick had the honors that day. Megan walked into the room and asked where my parents were. I told her they were in the waiting room. She told Patrick to go get them. I was so nervous. Was she going to tell me I wasn't in remission and wanted me to have the extra support?

Once everyone was seated, Megan told us the results had come back and I was in remission. She didn't have the written report yet, so it wasn't official, but as far as she was concerned, I was in remission. My tenderhearted dad had to wipe his tears. I sat there stunned while Patrick and Mom cheered. He did it! God answered the prayers of my loyal army. I had achieved remission after one round of chemo, thanks be to God.

After hearing the wonderful news, we began to make plans to go home. I was going to get about ten days of freedom. I asked Megan if I could work while I was home. She looked at me like I was nuts. I quickly told her I would just do three hours a day, and I would just stay in the office and not go in the field. She reluctantly agreed. My coworkers thought I was crazy too! But what no one realized was that I needed a normal routine to feel normal. I knew it would only be a few days, but it would be a few days I could pretend not to be sick.

The day I had been waiting for arrived! We were on the plane and going home. I was so excited I could hardly contain myself. I was sitting next to a man whom I had observed to be quite the jerk before we had even boarded the plane. He was so full of himself and was telling two young men where they needed to go and what they needed to do on their first trip to Alaska. One of his biggest pieces of advice was that these young men absolutely had to go to a famous Alaskan strip club. It was all I could do to keep quiet.

When I realized he was going to be my seat partner, I inwardly groaned. I decided I would just ignore him. But then he turned to me and asked, "It's obvious something is wrong with you—what do you have?" I guess the hat with no hair underneath clued him in. I told him I had recently been diagnosed with leukemia. He proceeded to tell me about all the members in his family who had recently died of cancer. Yep, I was sure feeling relaxed and normal.

We finally landed in Anchorage and collected our luggage. Dad looked at us and said, "Who is picking you up?" We evidently hadn't communicated well, as we had thought he and my mother were giving us a ride home. Unfortunately, Dad had his little two-seater truck at the airport. We decided we would make it work. Since I get extremely carsick, we all knew I had to sit in one of the two seats. Mom decided Patrick should drive. So, that left my parents to crawl in the little area behind the front two seats. I wish I had taken a picture of them. What they wouldn't do for love!

When they dropped us off, our dogs attacked me with kisses. Ringo, my rescued cattle-dog-mix boy, cried like a little baby. His mommy had been gone for six weeks, and he must have thought I was never coming back to him. I spent the afternoon puttering around the house, cleaning out the refrigerator and doing laundry. I napped on the couch with Ringo curled up at my feet. I woke up to Meghan and Kirk coming in with Olivienne. We were going to get to babysit! I closed my eyes for a moment and pretended everything was normal. I was so happy to be home.

Shortly after my diagnosis, our friend Paul had shipped our car to us. We had known Paul for several years, and he was a wonderful, Christian man. It was a kind and generous thing for him to do. Because my car was in Idaho, I had no car to drive while home. Granny offered the use of hers. Due to recent surgery, she wasn't driving anyway. I had planned just to relax on Friday and visit with Granny and family. I got a ride to her house and was welcomed with a big hug. Granny and I are very close, and it had been hard on both of us to be apart. After visiting with her, I decided to drop by the office and let my coworkers know I would be working on Monday. I was greeted with hugs and good wishes for my recovery. Everyone exclaimed at how good I looked in my wig. I was thrilled to be back.

At that time, I had thought I could go home a week each month to work. Unfortunately, I later found out that wasn't going to happen. I threw myself a couple of parties while I was home. There was an open invitation to all my friends and family to come visit. I was happy I got to see as many people as I did. Unfortunately, it was flu season in Alaska, so many had to stay away due to my compromised immune system. It was a great ten days. I loved being at work, I was happy to spend times with my kids, family, and friends, and we spent three glorious nights at our cabin over Thanksgiving.

Too soon my furlough was up. It was time to return to jail…But this time I had a new "cellie"! The wonderful owners of the Idaho house were allowing me to bring Ringo with me! I felt guilty about leaving Chester, our mastiff mix, but I was allowed one dog, and Ringo was my baby. Casey and Kelsey promised to take good care of Chester and our cat, Oreo. I packed my suitcase and tried to be brave as I said good-bye to my house, animals, family, and friends.

Twenty-One

TIME FOR ROUND TWO

Since I'd had my echocardiogram and heart ultrasound before
we left for home, we could get right down to business. We
drove to Post Falls clinic and got my poison pills. I wondered how
long I had before it hit me. We had dinner and went to the movies to see *Dumb and Dumber 2*. I started to feel sick just before the
movie ended but didn't say anything to Patrick until it was over.
Why worry him?

The next day I was feeling okay, so we decided to drive to Missoula,
Montana. I was in the mood for a road trip, and it wasn't as if we had
anything else to do! A big bonus for me was the Cracker Barrel restaurant I was going to get to go to. While Patrick drove, I tried to stay
awake and see the sights. I confess there were a few times that I dozed
off. First Stop—Cracker Barrel! We had a nice lunch, and I ate most
of my food. We then decided to explore the town.

Patrick isn't much of a "city guy," but he knows I judge a town by
its downtown area, so he humored me and drove around. Patrick

loves to find a body of water and dream about the fish that may be in there. We found Kelly's Landing, so of course we had to go! We were eager to explore a trail we found. We started out walking, but soon I realized it was time to take the poison pills. We swallowed our disappointment and walked back to the car. A short time later, I was sick, so we headed back to Idaho.

The next day I was very sick and exhausted, but I was determined to go back to Newport, Washington, to see Jim. Ringo and I took a long walk in the woods as soon as we got there. I tried visiting with Jim after my walk, but I was so tired. I went downstairs and fell asleep on his couch. What a load of fun I was! Patrick woke me up, I said good-bye to Jim, and off we went. The following day was day four—hospital admittance. I was supposed to be at the hospital early in the morning to get my new PICC line put in. Patrick was sleeping soundly, and I didn't want to wake him. I was feeling good, so I decided just to walk the mile and a half. I left my suitcase for him to bring over later. I knew he would be not be pleased with my decision, but it was a valid stand for my independence.

They had a hard time getting the PICC line in. My veins kept collapsing. When they hooked me up to the IV chemo, I felt sick again. Thank goodness for antinausea meds! When Patrick arrived, I had to endure a thirty-minute lecture about walking to the hospital alone. He loves me…

On day five, I walked sixty minutes and did forty-five squats, forty wall push-ups, and sixty arm raises with weights. I was not going to let the poison or Leuk win. Mom and our friend Gary were both there, and it was just one big party! Well, in between naps anyway. I wasn't sleeping at night because there was an elderly man across the hall yelling and crying all night long. He was scared and all alone. I wanted to visit him, but he possibly had Methicillin-resistant Staphylococcus aureus (MRSA), which is caused by a type of staph bacteria. There was no way I could go into his room. I wrote him a long letter of encouragement, and one of the staff members read it to him. The yelling didn't stop, so I broke down and asked to be moved to a new room. Lucky for me I got the remodeled room! It was the nicest room I had been in on One North.

Patrick and Gary brought Ringo to the hospital to see me. He wasn't allowed past the entryway, so Tad and I walked down the hall toward the door. When Ringo saw me, he started jumping up and down and crying. The poor dog had to be so confused. A couple and another woman at the door had observed Ringo's reaction and were touched by his devotion to me. They introduced themselves. Gene, his wife Leslie, and his sister Kathy had been visiting their mother. We got to talking about Alaska, and they wrote down their number and asked us to call if we needed anything at all. The next day they came to see me. They brought a huge tray of goodies, treats for Ringo, and a Walmart gift card! We were amazed at the kindness of strangers.

A friend of mine, who is a probation officer in Dillingham, Alaska, had asked his friend Reeva to come visit me. Reeva had never met me, but here she came with another friend and brought me an artificial Christmas tree. She lent me her iPod after discovering I didn't have one. We felt loved and blessed. I believe God sends people to those who need encouragement and comfort.

Patrick left for home on the seventh, and I later found out I got to leave that night! I was excited to get out of there. Casey sent me a text that really encouraged me. He told me how proud he was of me and encouraged me to continue the fight. Mom and I finally got to leave the hospital about nine o'clock. There was no way I was staying another night. I couldn't wait to escape.

The next day I was feeling very weak. I had an appointment to see one of my nurse practitioners, Jo, in the Coeur d'Alene clinic. I curled up in a chair in the waiting room. The CNA saw me and took me back to a room. She brought me a pillow and a blanket, and I stretched out on the examination table. Jo took one look at me and said, "You are going back into the hospital." I yelled, "No, please, no! I will be fine!"

She sent me upstairs to the infusion room, where they pumped me full of fluids. It didn't make a difference. The next day I felt the same. On top of it all, my arm was bruised and swollen where the PICC line was inserted. It had to come out. I had no choice but to go back to the hospital. They tried to wheel me over in a wheelchair, but I refused. If I had to go back, I would go on my terms. I hadn't lost my stubborn streak. I had never let them wheel me anywhere while in the hospital. During my first hospital stay, they had showed up with a gurney to take me to x-ray. I threw a fit, and Casey told me I was acting like Olivienne. Okay, maybe I was a little stubborn, but I wasn't going to give in to Leuk! I would fight him as hard as I could.

My medical team was concerned that I had a blood clot in my arm from the PICC. Ironically, while I was being checked for that, my little cousin Chelsey was in intensive care in an Anchorage hospital for a blood clot in her leg. I thought about her constantly and asked my faithful warriors to pray for her too. It was so hard to be so far away, in separate hospitals, for the same thing. I felt so bad for Granny. I knew she was extremely worried about both her granddaughters.

After two days and a clear CT scan, they released me. Chelsey remained in the hospital, and I felt guilty for being able to leave when she couldn't. Two days later, my arm was still the same. My PA, Megan, sent me to the hospital for an ultrasound. I was afraid I would be readmitted. She later called me and told me they had found a clot, but it was small, and they weren't worried. I escaped incarceration! Besides giving me the good news about the clot, she told me the Mayo Clinic had finally responded to the e-consult; I did not need a transplant. Hallelujah, thank you, Lord! It was the one thing I had been absolutely terrified about. I was terribly afraid of repeating Logan's experience. We had watched him suffer daily, and I didn't want my family to go through it again. After all he had gone through, he had succumbed to a fungal infection. I figured the same thing would happen to me. I was glad to hear Plan A was going to work.

The following day Mom and I drove to Cheney, Washington, to go to a live Nativity event with my friend Faith and her family. It was a beautiful event, and we were glad to get out of the house and away from medical facilities. Despite the fun time with Mom and friends, I was lamenting the fact I was not in Alaska attending a retirement party we had planned to go to for the last year. I had been so excited about it and was sad Patrick was there without me. He called me later and told me I was missed by everyone. I just wanted to go home.

• • •

My dad was coming to see me, and I was so excited! I noticed a bunch of bruises on my legs the morning he was to arrive. I figured I might need some platelets, but I felt good. When I was brushing my teeth, I noticed weird black marks on my tongue and the inside of my cheeks. They looked like blood blisters. I called the clinic and was told that Jo would look at them during my scheduled appointment that day. Mom and I had a bet on what my platelet level was.

I still felt well, so I went on a long walk with Ringo. Mom went to pick Dad up from the airport. I missed the text Dad sent me telling me they would be back in time to drive me to my appointment. I was still full of energy, so I decided to walk the mile and a half to the clinic. I had been walking about fifteen minutes when I realized that probably wasn't the best idea I had ever had. I was out of breath and had to keep stopping to rest. Dad called me to ask where I was. I had taken a different path and couldn't give very good directions. I assured him I was fine, but inside I wasn't so sure I was going to make it there. When I was almost there, I chose to run across the street at a busy intersection because I didn't want to walk another fifty feet to the crosswalk. I ended up utilizing more energy than I would have if I had just walked the extra feet.

When I got to the door, my parents were waiting for me with their arms crossed and disapproval written all over their faces. Dad said, "I don't know whether to spank you or hug you!" I told him my platelets were probably low, so he better just hug me. I had to listen to the parental lecture for several minutes. It was nice to be loved.

I had my blood drawn, and we waited for the results. When Jo walked in, I stuck my tongue out at her and asked her what the heck was wrong with me. She laughed and said, "You need platelets immediately; you are down to three thousand." The normal range for platelets is 150,000 to 300,000. I was dangerously low. On top of that, my hemoglobin was also extremely low. She told me I would likely need red blood cells the following day. Walking over four miles that day may not have been the wisest thing to do, but by gosh, I did it! The next day Patrick arrived in time for my red blood cell transfusion.

Twenty-Two

CHRISTMAS AND NEW YEAR'S EVE FOR TWO, PLEASE

Since Mom and Dad were leaving before Christmas, we decided to have an early Christmas dinner. Mom made a delicious dinner of ham and scalloped potatoes, and we invited our friend Jan over. For the first time in our entire married lives, we were going to be alone on Christmas Day. On the eighteenth, we dropped Mom and Dad off at the Holiday Lights Cruise. They had a special night planned for them by their grandchildren. Meghan and Kirk had bought them tickets for the cruise, and Casey and Kelsey had paid for them to stay in a bed-and-breakfast close by. With all the traveling back and forth, along with their insane schedule at home, they were overdue for a break. I was happy they were going to get some time alone.

I wanted to get some Christmas shopping done even though my counts weren't sufficient to fight off infections. We certainly couldn't do much purchasing that year, but there were a few things I wanted to get. While Patrick was driving, I turned my head and pretended to be looking out the window. I had tears streaming down my face, and I felt an overwhelming feeling of sadness and despair. I was sure this was going to be my last Christmas. I wondered if he would get remarried and if he would still love me if he had a new wife. Would my children tell their children about me? Would the kids even miss someone they never got to know? As Patrick parked the car, I quickly wiped my tears and put on a happy face. I was tired and worn out, but I refused to show how badly I felt physically and emotionally.

The next night I had two disturbing dreams of abandoning Logan. I assumed they had something to do with the guilt that I had because he had died and I was trying to live. For years, I would have welcomed death because the pain of losing a child was so debilitating. But now I had a renewed desire to remain with my family. My work wasn't over; there were so many people I wanted to help. I wanted to be a good mother to my children, and I wanted to be the best grammie I could be to Olivienne and my future grandchildren. I wanted to be married to the man I loved, who had stood beside me. I didn't want my parents, grandma, and family to suffer any more losses.

Besides the emotional pain I was experiencing, I felt terrible physically. I started running a fever. It would go up, then down, and back up again. It never reached the point where I had to be admitted, and I was thankful for that. I wondered if this was ever going to end.

Mom left on Christmas Eve, and Dad had left a couple days prior. I wasn't feeling well, so I stayed home while Patrick took her to the airport in Spokane. I didn't tell either one that I was running a fever again. I texted Casey and Mindy and swore them to secrecy. I guess I thought that if no one knew, it wouldn't go up. Casey told me he would be praying hard that it would go down. Mindy kept telling me I needed to call my doctor. For hours, it would creep up and then hold steady. I finally called the on-call doctor, Dr. Kim, and asked him if I could just take some Tylenol, and he agreed. When I told Patrick about taking Tylenol, he lectured me about "doctor shopping." Dr. Mulvey had warned me not to mask my symptoms by taking Tylenol. I didn't care; I was fever-free and not going to be in the hospital on Christmas Day.

On Christmas Day I wasn't feeling that great, but I felt better as the day went on. We took Ringo for a walk, and I saw people climbing Tubbs Hill. I declared we were going to do that! Patrick tried to discourage me. He knew how competitive I was and worried I would be disappointed if I didn't make it up. I assured him I would be okay with turning around if I needed to. I had to stop several times due to breathing issues, but we made it to the end of the trail! Granted, we stayed on the main trail and didn't do a ton of extreme climbing, but I did it! Success was mine. Die, Leuk, die!

Not only did I complete a physically challenging climb, but I had something else to look forward to. Meghan was coming with Olivienne. We had the pleasure of their company from the twenty-sixth to the thirtieth. How wonderful it was to see them both! I was so grateful that Meghan was willing to come with the baby each month. When home, Olivienne would sleep about ten hours each night. While in Idaho, she kept her momma up most nights. It was a huge sacrifice for Meghan, and I appreciated it so much. Since I have always been an early riser, Ollie and I settled into a routine. She would whimper early in the morning, and Grammie would rush in and pick her up. Ollie entertained us the entire time.

Too soon the visited ended, and we took them to the airport. It was so hard to say good-bye. I cried all the way back to Coeur d'Alene. How could I be a part of Ollie's life when I could only see her one week each month? My only consolation was realizing she did remember me each time she visited. Patrick took me to Red Lobster and bribed me with biscuits in hopes that I would be cheerful again.

As the year was ending, I reflected on my many blessings. Despite being diagnosed with leukemia and having multiple transfusions, strange rashes, multiple central lines, and nausea from treatment, I had a good life. We had been blessed by so many people. We had many visits from people we knew who were in the area and took the time to see us. Some came specifically to see us, including one of my closest friends, Pam, who lives in Germany. Each visit was a gift to me; I was loved. The blessings were abundant. We had been blessed with meals from a local church group, our car was shipped from Alaska for free, and we were offered a beautiful house to stay in. We were given financial support to help with costs. Our employers and coworkers were amazing, and my dog got to be with me. In the darkness of the storm, I saw the light of Jesus shining through so many people. It was a humbling experience to rely on others, but God orchestrated it all.

I was supposed to start round three of chemo on the thirtieth of December. I had begged my medical team to let me start on the second so that I wouldn't be sick over New Year's Eve. On the thirtieth, I had to get my labs done. I was still neutropenic, and my platelets were still low, so I couldn't have started anyway. I wasn't concerned, as I was sure they would soon be up.

New Year's Eve was like what we experienced in Alaska; I fell asleep early. I was hoping it would be different that year. I woke up just before midnight and watched the firework display from our front window. What mattered most was I was alive and out of the hospital, and Patrick and I were together. The next day I wanted to go on a road trip—this time to Canada! We grabbed our passports, camera, and dog and headed out. It took us about an hour and a half to reach the border. The border patrol officer asked where we were from. Patrick replied that we were from Coeur d'Alene. He then asked why we were driving a car with Alaska plates. Patrick explained we were really from Alaska but temporarily living in Coeur d'Alene. I realized he would never say I was being treated for leukemia when someone asked why we were in Idaho. I think he wanted to keep that to himself. If he didn't say it out loud, it wasn't true. My heart hurt for him.

The officer continued to ask questions. "What's your destination in Canada? What will you be doing? How long will you be here?"

Patrick replied, "We don't know where we are going to go, not sure what we are going to do, and probably will be here for a couple of hours."

The border patrol officer looked at us in disbelief as he said, "You are only staying a couple of hours? Why?" Patrick shrugged and replied that we were just out for a drive. I hung my head and thought, "He's either going to arrest us because he thinks we are drug dealers, or he's going to tell us to turn around and go back to Idaho." To my surprise, he waved us through.

Our next carefree adventure had begun. I pretended that we were just on vacation and out for an adventure. I tried not to think about the next round of chemo. We were just a normal couple out for a short drive in Canada. We decided to turn on the road toward Creston. The terrain looked like Alaska, and we felt at home. We arrived in Creston about forty-five minutes later. It looked like a ghost town. Most of the shops were closed, and hardly any people were strolling about. Of course, it was New Year's Day, and most places were closed. I didn't think that excursion out very well.

We found a hotel that had a pub inside. At least we could have food. We had a nice lunch and then drove around a bit. Soon it was time to head back to the border. We saw a sign in Creston that said, "This way to the USA border." We thought about taking it, but that wasn't the way we had come, and we weren't sure where we would end up. Besides I had seen a couple of cool bridges I wanted to take pictures of. We headed back the way we had come. When we got to the border, it was a repeat of our earlier experience. This officer was suspicious of why we were in Canada for two hours and why we didn't take the border crossing from Creston. I figured our visits to Canada were numbered: we were suspected dealers. We had a good laugh about it and headed back to Idaho.

Twenty-Three

Unwanted News

January 18, 2015…I think this day was harder on me then October 11, 2014, the day I was diagnosed. The day started off well. Mom and I did a water-aerobics class together. Mom was always willing to try new things. She was a great person to hang out with. We shared lots of laughs, but there was something hanging over our heads, and we couldn't fully relax.

I had been trying to start round three since the beginning of January. My spirits were up and I was ready, but my body wouldn't cooperate. I was still neutropenic. My ANC had to be one thousand and my platelets had to be fifty thousand. For days, my numbers barely budged. To top it off, I was really dehydrated. Megan said I needed IV fluids. A sweet nurse named Erin made three attempts to start an IV. Each attempt resulted in my veins being infiltrated, which meant the fluids were going into my surrounding tissues rather than my veins. My arm and hands swelled up. After the third attempt, I reassured Erin it wasn't her fault, but I would not sit there and try again. I would drink the bag of saline if I had to.

A few days later, despite the increase in fluids, my dehydration issues had not resolved. Another attempt was made to start an IV. No luck. One of the most experienced nurses in the clinic was unable to find a vein. Again, I said no more. That night I drank two gallons of fluids. My counts were still low. The next day when I went into the clinic, I had dressed in a Wonder Woman hat and jacket. Dr. Mulvey took one look at me and said, "What on earth are you wearing?" I told him I was wearing my WW outfit to bring me strength and make my numbers go up. He told me it didn't work.

Megan and Dr. Mulvey told me I needed another bone marrow biopsy to see if I had relapsed. It was my third bone marrow biopsy since October. They were in a hurry, and the procedure was done almost immediately. I was told the preliminary results would be back the following day. We waited anxiously by the phone. Finally, about 4:25 p.m., Dr. Mulvey called to tell me it looked good! The final report wouldn't be ready until Monday, but he was encouraged; there was no increase in blasts. Oh, how we celebrated! Plan A would continue!

Unfortunately, our celebration came to a quick end a couple days later. Dr. Mulvey called to tell me I had relapsed after all. I had about 15 percent blasts in my marrow. He said, "It doesn't look good. You have about a 40 percent chance of going into remission, and you have to have a bone marrow transplant." He asked me if I wanted to do the repeat of induction here or at the Mayo Clinic. My head was spinning. He wanted me to decide right then? I wasn't ready to leave Idaho. I was comfortable with my medical team. I told him I wanted to do the induction in Coeur d'Alene. As hard as this was on me, it didn't compare to how hard it was on my family.

My mom shed many tears as I sat there numbly in disbelief. I had wanted Plan A. I had believed Plan A would happen. I prayed, "What is your plan, Lord? Show me, please. Show my family because they are hurting. Don't let me doubt or lose my faith. Don't leave me, Jesus." All I could think was, "I will fight to live, but if I die, I know where I am going. It's the ones left behind who hurt the most." Despite my sorrow and despair, this was nothing compared to watching my son die.

From the start, I felt Mayo Clinic was the best place to go if I needed a transplant. We earnestly began searching for places to live in Rochester, Minnesota, where Mayo Clinic is. That's where I was treated for osteomyelitis when I was twelve. I had stayed in Saint Mary's Hospital for almost a month. It's a nice town, but what was most important was the wonderful reputation Mayo Clinic had. I wanted the best, because I wanted to live. From the beginning, I refused to go to Seattle. Logan was treated in Seattle and had died after his transplant. We didn't have very many good memories of Seattle. Seattle was closer to home, though, and it was close to the headquarters of Patrick's employers, and we had friends there. What place was the best place for me? I sure didn't know. I just wanted to live. On top of trying to stay alive, I had to worry about my job and insurance. I didn't know what was going to happen with me being gone for so long. There were so many things to consider. I asked for prayers to know what the right path for me was and prayers to stomp Leuk into the ground and send him back to hell where he belonged.

Dr. Mulvey called to tell us Mayo Clinic wanted to see us right away. They could do chemo there, but I wasn't ready to leave Idaho. I wanted to regroup—to go home while the search for a donor was implemented. The upcoming round of chemo was going to be rough, and I was told to expect to be in the hospital for a month. I had to go back to the clinic to get labs drawn. My arm swelled up immediately when Todd put the needle in. I confess I cried. Not because it hurt, but because it seemed my body was failing me. I felt so good, so how could I be so sick? My white count didn't go up at all, but my platelets did. Dr. Mulvey told me that soon all my levels would drop. Without chemo, I would die. They had to get me in remission and keep me there before the transplant. The target goal for transplant was in the month of April.

There were many moments where I was simply confused. I flashed back to a memory of Pastor Dennis Hotchkiss speaking at Logan's funeral. He said his daughter Haley kept saying, "Daddy, I am confused. Why did Logan die? We prayed for him. I am confused." I was also confused as to why Logan had died when we had so much faith. And I was confused when I relapsed as well. I tried so hard and was so hopeful. My hopefulness turned to disappointment. "What is your master plan, God?" I asked. I was looking at the current circumstances but couldn't understand the big picture. There were twists and turns at every corner, just as there had been on the road with Logan. From my limited perspective, there was confusion. But from God's perspective, there was a plan: "And we know that for those who love God, all things work together for good, for those who are called according to his purpose" (Rom. 8:28).

I didn't claim to have the answer as to why my family was going through this again. I couldn't explain why Logan had died after receiving a bone marrow transplant when we and hundreds, maybe thousands, had prayed faithfully for him. I couldn't explain why God had allowed me to contract leukemia and then relapse when we thought everything was going so well. I couldn't explain why I had to face my fears of reliving Logan's transplant by having my own. What I did know was that every last breath I had would be spent thanking my Lord for loving me and dying for me so that I might live in eternity with him. Yes, I was afraid of what was to come, but I also had the peace of a personal relationship with my God. I was in a win-win situation. I would fight to remain on this earth. But if God chose for me to leave this earth early, I would accept it.

Twenty-Four

WONDER WOMAN'S SUPPORT TEAM ROCKS

The support I received from friends and family was simply unbelievable. I went from being scared and feeling alone to feeling like I had a mighty army behind me. The power in numbers was amazing. I couldn't imagine going into a battlefield without many trained soldiers standing beside me. My army of soldiers was ready to battle with me; I was not alone. I wasn't sure why so many loved and supported me, but I was so thankful. Patrick and my mom took turns being the general and helping me make the difficult decisions. Being a frugal person who doesn't like to spend money on myself, I found it difficult to imagine what I was costing my family. Patrick put it this way: "We are not pinching pennies and buying medicine at Walmart! You will get the best care, no matter what the cost is."

In my gut, I felt Mayo Clinic was the best place for me. I tried putting my feelings about Seattle aside, but every time I thought about having my transplant there, I got sick to my stomach. Logically it was the best place, but it just didn't feel right.

Patrick flew back to Idaho on January 20. I was so thankful to have him there with me. He had a way of making everything seem okay. He has always been an optimistic person. I used to get irritated hearing him say, "It will all work out okay" when I was concerned about something. But during these trying times, his words were music to my ears. Mom and I continued our workouts and even did two back-to-back water-aerobics classes one day. We danced around the pool and pretended nothing was wrong. I was determined to continue getting stronger.

There were moments that made me question whether we had made the right decision to go to Mayo. The process to get an appointment was simply a nightmare. Whoever answered the phone in the hematology/oncology clinic told me Dr. Mulvey had told her I couldn't come for an evaluation. I assured her that was not the case and we needed an appointment right away. She told me the first appointment available was February 18. My heart seemed to stop. I told her if I didn't start chemo soon I would likely die. She said that was the best she could do.

I hung up and called my doctor's office. Shannon promised Dr. Mulvey would get it straightened out. Just after I hung up with her, the woman from Mayo Clinic called back and said they had a cancelation for tomorrow. I told her I couldn't possibly go tomorrow because I had family coming in and still had to buy tickets. She informed me she would let Dr. Hogan know I had refused the appointment. I admit my resolve was shaken. I felt abandoned and left alone to figure it out on my own. It was too much to handle!

Thankfully, Dr. Mulvey straightened it out. Another (more efficient) woman called me back and told me my first appointment would be on Tuesday. I needed to be there for three days. I was to have multiple tests done, including a psychological exam. At that moment, I didn't feel so mentally sound. One minute I was happy as could be, and the next minute I was crying.

I spent the afternoon trying to buy tickets, get the insurance paperwork completed, and so on. I went to the library and checked out a couple of books. The librarian said, "These are due back in two weeks." I thanked her and walked out wondering if my doctors would tell me I just had a couple of weeks to live. What if the chemo didn't work, and I failed to go back into remission? I remembered Logan's doctor telling us he had just a short time to live. I wanted to throw something. I ran crying from the room. We never told Logan he was going to die. I didn't want to scare him. But I was an adult, and I needed to know so I could say good-bye.

Twenty-Five

GATHERING TOGETHER AS ONE

When bad news was shared, my family came running. I was so excited when Meghan and Olivienne flew down. Olivienne ran to me with open arms at the airport. That was the definition of happiness. Having her remember me was such an amazing feeling, and it helped me hold on to hope during difficult times. My parents were simply the best grandparents for my three children, and I wanted to be the best grammie for Olivienne.

How I missed those lunch hours when I would go see Ollie and Meghan. I loved getting my baby hugs. Sometimes Meghan would meet me at work, and we would spend my lunch hour walking together. It's funny how easy it is for people to take spending time with family and friends for granted. How many times have you thought about getting together with someone you care about, only to dismiss the idea because you were too busy? I know I have. I learned to savor every moment I had with those I loved.

One morning, Patrick and I took Ollie and Ringo to the dog park. Ollie had more fun playing on the dog equipment than Ringo did. Ringo just wanted to sit beside me on the bench. We enjoyed being together and laughed a lot. Olivienne wasn't crazy about her stroller, so Patrick and I took turns carrying her. It wasn't long before I was gasping for air. My strength had greatly diminished.

My dad arrived the following day. If you want to draw attention to yourself and have everyone cater to you, get diagnosed with leukemia! I sure missed my dad. He wrapped his arms around me and told me we were going to give it all we had. He told me we would beat this stupid cancer. I trusted my dad, and I knew he was right. As we both said, it wasn't going to be easy, but we would make it through.

Not only did I worry about what was ahead, but I was still concerned about our finances. Last-minute airfare to Minnesota was outrageously expensive, and I wasn't sure how we were going to be able to afford it. Thanks to a very generous woman named Connie, however, we had enough money to pay for our plane tickets to Mayo Clinic as well as our hotel and rental car. We attended the same church as Connie for many years. She and her husband, Steve, were a great couple, and I really liked them both. Steve had recently died after a hard battle with cancer. We appreciated her generosity so much. I think blessing us financially was a way to honor her husband. I can't say enough about our community during this time. Fundraisers and bone marrow drives were being planned, and we were humbled and grateful. We were simply amazed at the generosity of so many people.

Before we left for Mayo, we had an appointment with my PA, Megan. Mom, Patrick, and Meghan were with me while Dad babysat Ollie. Megan went over the plan for chemo. I was very concerned because I hadn't had chemotherapy since the beginning of December. Of course, I worried that the blasts cells would increase even more, which would make a second remission more difficult to achieve. I wanted to put my head in the sand and pretend everything was okay. I didn't want to talk about hospitalizations, treatment, or blood counts. I wanted to decide what day worked best for babysitting and what I was going to do in my lunch hour. I wanted to be normal.

I saw the sadness in Megan's eyes when she told me she was sorry I had relapsed. I was doing well until she asked how I was doing. I had to fight back the tears as I told her I was okay. We discussed our upcoming appointment at Mayo, anticipated time frames for chemo, and what to expect. I was told that the next round would likely be very difficult with more chances of having mouth sores, infections, and transfusions. There was a possibility that I wouldn't have any increased issues, though. I wasn't going to fret about it.

We were not looking forward to starting over with new providers, a new city, and a new hospital. We found each person we had contact with in Coeur d'Alene to be genuinely compassionate. Everyone knew us by name, remembered details, and treated us as friends rather than as just another patient.

Blood tests were done frequently in the days before we left for Mayo Clinic. I was nervous about getting my blood drawn again because of the swelling in my arms. I didn't understand why the body I had always taken such good care of was failing me. How could it betray me like that? Despite my disappointment that Leuk had returned and was trying to destroy me, I never once stopped and asked, "Why me?" Now I understand how Logan had felt. He was so sick after his transplant, and it had been unbearable to watch my baby suffer.

One day I had broken down crying and said, "It's not fair you have to go through this." He had responded by saying, "Mom, it's not fair that anyone has to go through this." He was eleven then. What an amazing boy! There wasn't a selfish or self-centered bone in his body. I felt like Logan did. It's not fair that anyone must suffer. I would not wish this on someone else instead. I'm no better than anyone else, so why not me?

The following day was amazing! I had my parents, my husband, our daughter, and our grandchild with me. We laughed and savored every moment we had. We attempted to take Ollie swimming at the fitness center but didn't realize no children were allowed in the pool on Tuesdays and Thursdays. Ollie was content to just run around. Meghan decided to work out, and we were going to babysit. I felt utterly exhausted. Despite my disappointment, I let Patrick talk me into going back to the house to rest while he hung out with Olivienne. It was hard to accept my limitations. I felt completely inept as a grandmother. Ollie didn't think I was inept, though! Much to my delight, Olivienne wanted her grammie a lot. She wanted me to carry her around, hugged me, and gave me lots of kisses. It was an amazing feeling to be loved by the most adorable baby in the world!

After my nap, Meghan said we should go back to the fitness center and sit in the outdoor tub. I thought about it for a second and then said, "You know what? I'm tired of not being spontaneous anymore. Let's do it!" Mom wasn't sure the heat would be a good idea, nor did she want me around a lot of people. Dad said he wouldn't go because I might embarrass him. I had been telling stories about almost losing my bikini top in water aerobics, and he just wasn't sure what we wild and crazy girls might do! We took off and went for it.

The night was cold, and it was snowing. I left my shirt on over my swimsuit as we headed outside for the hot tub. I always wore two hats: a thin one and then a knitted one on top. I took off my shirt, and the knitted one fell off in the pool. I laid my shirt and towel down, and we proceeded to get into the very warm tub. Meghan and I talked about my treatment, delaying Ollie's immunizations for my safety, questions we had about my upcoming treatment, and just general topics—whatever came to mind. My daughter loved me so much, and she must have been so scared thinking she might lose her mom. She had a friend who had recently lost her mother to cancer, and I know Meghan thought about her a lot. She was a lot like her grandmother; she remained so brave and matter-of-fact. Those two women anchored me, for sure!

When we got out of the hot tub, we realized that not only was the hat that fell in wet, but so were my towel and shirt! Oh, I hadn't thought that one out very well. But then neither had Meghan. She had not even brought a towel. We had a good laugh at our "well-thought-out plan." Oh well, we were spontaneous!

The next day I had to have another ultrasound on my arm because the swelling from the blood draw had never gone away. They determined it was not deep vein thrombosis, just a hematoma. I also got good news about my six-month checkup for HIV and Hep C. Both came back negative—thank you, God! I was told that was the final test I needed for both diseases. The last thing I needed was to hear I was positive for another thing.

I got a surprise visit from my brother, sister-in-law, and two nieces. They flew from Anchorage to spend just one night with me. Things were looking up, and I felt so loved by so many. The joy of being with my family boosted my spirits and helped give me courage for the long road ahead. I don't know how anyone could get through cancer treatment without the support of family and friends.

The visit with my brother and his family went way too fast. How could I possibly be content with a one-day visit when I was used to seeing them several times a week? I learned to make the most out of short visits, though. We took a long walk together before they left. As usual, Sharmin, Melissa, and I left the rest in the dust. We didn't realize how far we had gotten ahead until we stopped at an intersection. I felt relieved that I could continue at such a great pace all the way back to the house. However, it wasn't long before I was exhausted and ready to curl up and go to sleep. I couldn't miss out on a single moment with them, though. Nap time would have to wait.

We went out for pizza, and I sat quietly at the table soaking in the love of my family. I felt blessed beyond belief. Saying good-bye wasn't easy. My strong brother, who has always been someone I have admired, broke down and cried as he held on to me as if it would be the last time he saw me. I know none of us know the exact moment we are going to die. But I can tell you that knowing

I had a life-threatening illness made me appreciate my family, friends, and everything around me more. Colors seemed brighter, rain didn't bother me, and I loved my family and friends more than ever. Little things didn't matter anymore.

I was nervous and apprehensive for what was to come. We had struck Leuk down so quickly the first round. But he was stronger than I had thought. I had believed him to be a weak adversary, but unfortunately, he had decided to be my nemesis. But my faith could move mountains.

Twenty-Six

Trip to Mayo Clinic

I had trouble sleeping the night before we left. I woke up several times wondering what I would hear. Would the doctors at the Mayo Clinic tell me they were my best option? Or would they say they couldn't help me? What if they said there was no hope? All those thoughts swarmed my mind as I attempted to sleep.

It was hard to say good-bye to Meghan and Olivienne. It was never easy giving them that last hug knowing it might be a while before I would see them again. I knew I might be too sick to see Ollie the next time I saw her. I kept reminding myself of this verse: "Therefore do not be anxious about tomorrow, for tomorrow will be anxious for itself. Sufficient for the day is its own trouble" (Matt. 6:34).

We were ready to face the man who held my future in his medical hands. What was he going to say? Would he give us hope? I couldn't escape the apprehension no matter how hard I tried. For someone who usually had every moment of her life planned, it was a true testament to being patient and letting God take the wheel. I knew I would be able to go with the flow as soon as I had a plan. But at that moment, all I could do was wonder when I would be returning to the prison to resume getting poison to kill Leuk. Leuk needed to die, but since my body was his host, I too would be punished when the poison was injected into my body.

Wonder Woman never hesitated to put her life on the line for the good of humanity. I refused to hesitate either. I was willing to fight with all I had to win the fierce battle. I envisioned my cells fighting inside my body. There were the good cells trying to fight off the bad cells. They waged a battle deep inside my marrow, and I knew the good guys must win.

Our first appointment at the Mayo Clinic went as planned. We met with Darci, the nurse practitioner, who answered most of our questions and explained some of the process. My counts looked good.

I was upset with the phlebotomist because she used a regular-sized needle and dug around attempting to find a vein, and it hurt. I had scar tissue built up on my left arm and a hematoma on my right. I didn't have much to choose from. She needed nine tubes of blood. I finally asked her nicely to take the needle out and use a smaller needle, which was referred to as a "butterfly." Patrick always told me I needed to be more vocal, but I never wanted to hurt anyone's feelings. He was right, though, and I worked on being politely assertive.

They also did my Human Leukocyte Antigen typing (HLA). HLA typing is done so they could compare my genes to the genes of people in the bone marrow registry in hopes of finding a match for me. The process had changed since we did the testing when Logan needed a transplant. Whereas earlier a blood test was used, it is now a simple swab of the inside of a person's cheek. I had to swish mouthwash around my mouth for twenty seconds. Instead of taking a little, I had about three-fourths of it in my mouth without realizing it. I was trying not to laugh as I mimed the motion I needed to spit some out. I followed it with swishing water for the same amount of time. The lab technician gave me very cold water, and we both tried not to laugh as I attempted to swish. After that she scrubbed both of my cheeks with a swab.

Dr. Hogan seemed very knowledgeable and agreed to allow me to return to Idaho for reinduction. He explained that I would have six days of very intensive chemo and would remain in the hospital until I was no longer neutropenic, which was expected to take about a month. A bone marrow biopsy would be done on day fourteen. I held on to this thought: "Wonder Woman is going to kick Leuk's ass! He is going down! I will throttle him and poison him. He will cry for mercy, but I will look at him with scorn and say, 'God and Wonder Woman have defeated you, you slime!'"

I had an appointment with a psychiatrist first thing in the morning. I hadn't slept well, and I was frustrated because I couldn't check my e-mail due to Hotmail issues. I was in the lobby for about forty minutes before I was even called back. I think they have a devious strategy in making people wait. They want to see how many lose their cool in the lobby. I was afraid that I would succumb to my rising level of frustration. But alas, I was called back before I completely gave in to my frustration. I met with a nurse the first hour. She asked me a series of questions and went over the questionnaire I had filled out. I don't think those questionnaires were right for someone in my situation. Yes, I was stressed and anxious, and yes, I was having trouble sleeping. Who wouldn't be if they had recently found out they had relapsed and needed a bone marrow transplant? I was physically and emotionally exhausted.

My favorite story about not sleeping was the time my overeager CNA came in at one o'clock in the morning to tell me she was hanging a paper on the door and that every time I went to the bathroom, I could write down how much urine there was. Then she wanted to know if I wanted to be weighed right then or wait until five o'clock. This was after I had made an agreement with my nurses that they would leave me alone for a few hours so I could sleep a bit. I refrained from throwing said urine at her.

After I met with the nurse, I was directed to return to the lobby and wait for the psychiatrist. She too stressed how important it was for me to sleep. I guess they had never been patients in a hospital before. The doctor wanted to talk about Logan's treatment and death and how I was dealing with being in a similar situation. I told her that it sucked and that I was really pissed off about it, but it is what it is and I would take one day at a time. I told her about my incredible support group and how our community was helping us.

My next appointment was with a social worker, and then we were given a couple of hours for a lunch break. I was feeling hungry, so we found a popular pizza restaurant. I went into the restroom to wash my hands. I glanced in the mirror and was disgusted at how bad I looked. I looked tired, drained, and old. I sat down across from Patrick and told him that when my hair came back, I would never wear another hat as long as I lived.

Twenty-Seven

Unbelievable News

We returned to the clinic to finish that day's testing. Just when we were about out the door, Darci, my nurse practitioner called. She said I needed to go back to the lab and have another blood draw. My heart nearly stopped as she told me my HIV test had come back positive. I had been tested several times after being stuck with the dirty needle. All results were negative. The last one was just done on January 23, exactly six months to the day since I was stuck with a needle used by a heroin addict. That test was negative. Now it came up positive?

I was listening to her and tried to get Patrick to wait. All he could think about was bringing the car up so I wouldn't have to walk out in the cold. He didn't hear my pleas to wait. I stood in that lobby and felt the sheer terror come over me. I was literally drowning in panic. Darci told me they believed it was a false positive, but they had to be sure. I walked like a zombie back through the maze of halls to the lab. I checked in again, choking back tears as I told her I was back for an HIV test.

I had a different phlebotomist. Was it my imagination, or did she treat me like I was some drug addict who was worth nothing? She was cold and uncaring as she too dug around in my arm to find a vein.

I got lost trying to find my way back to the lobby. I felt like I did when Logan died. I was confused, and nothing made sense. I looked up and saw Patrick standing there. I leaned against him and sobbed. How can this be? Hadn't I been punished enough? Why was this happening? It was bad enough that I had to go through the same process that had killed my firstborn son. But to possibly have HIV on top of leukemia? What a sick, cruel joke. Statistics show that fewer than 1 percent of people accidentally stuck with a dirty needle contract HIV. I took that horrible medication that is 99.7 percent successful in preventing HIV. The medicine that made me terribly sick. The medicine I was convinced caused my leukemia. The odds should have been in my favor.

Patrick tried to console me the best he could. After hours of grieving, I concluded there was nothing I could do to change the situation. I could be mad at God and the whole world, or I could face this with dignity, faith, and grace. I chose to trust my God even though I did not understand. Waiting with hope was very difficult. Waiting for hope took strength and patience, but my strength would only grow by waiting. I went back to a verse that frequently comforted me during this process, "Be of good courage and He shall strengthen your heart, all you who hope in the Lord" (Ps. 31:24).

Several days later, I got the news that once again God had intervened, and my HIV test was in fact negative. We were cleared for the next step.

Twenty-Eight

REINDUCTION SOON BEGINS

I checked into Kootenai Hospital in Coeur d'Alene, and an orderly took me to short stay to put PICC number three in. Ringo had to stay at the house in Coeur d'Alene. I tried to explain to him that Mommy had to go away for a while because she was sick. He looked at me like I was nuts. I told him, "I know I don't look sick; I don't feel sick either!" I was still in shock about all of this. How could I feel so good when cancer cells were running around my bone marrow? I kept thinking all the tests were wrong. Maybe just a little pill was all I needed to have more energy. The new chemo they would be giving me the next few days sounded awful. "No, thank you," I would love to have said. "You may keep your vomiting-inducing, mouth-sore inducing poison; I don't want it."

But alas, they connected me with Tad once again and planned to hold me hostage for days on end, filling me with horrible stuff that might kill Leuk. The only thing I had ever killed was a mosquito. I turned into a hunter; I declared that I would hunt the bastard down and slay him. How I despised Leuk! He had robbed me of my energy, my health, and my normal life. But he had not robbed me of my faith. He couldn't take away the love I had for my family and friends.

Despite my circumstances, I had such joy and delight being around the medical staff. As usual, I refused to get on a gurney or ride in a wheelchair. The regular escort guys remembered me, but I had two new ones who just didn't know what to think of me. A very young one named Zach told me he just couldn't let me walk because it was against policy. I told him they made exceptions for me. I felt sorry for the poor kid, but I wasn't budging. After he made the call and got approval, I walked to get my heart tests. The poor guy was so flustered that he forgot my chart on the gurney. He had to run back to get it. He brought it into the room where I was getting my echocardiogram and tried to lay it on the sink with his eyes averted. Heaven forbid if he saw me disrobed! He dropped the chart in the sink. Poor kid.

The technicians who put my PICC line in remembered me as the only one who had ever walked into their room dancing. They seemed disappointed that I didn't bring music for the procedure. Before I walked into their room, I talked my patient escort, Dillon, into getting on the gurney while I hid behind the door. I seemed to have a reputation, and I wasn't sure if that was good or bad.

I spent my time in the hospital visiting with many friends, playing games, and walking. The highlight of that stay was Super Bowl Sunday. I slept through most of the game, but Patrick and his friends didn't. They stayed at the house and drank beer while watching the game. Mom brought them back to the hospital after the game. The only problem was, they'd had just a little bit too much to drink. We decided to go for a walk in the halls, and it was all I could do to keep them quiet! Steve decided he wanted to play hide-and-go-seek, Patrick demanded I push him in a wheelchair while he sang "The Ants Go Marching In," and Dennis just happily floated around egging everyone on. I joined in on the festivities and jumped on top of a bench, proud that I still had moves. We just about got busted by a very stern-looking employee. The last thing I needed was to get kicked out of a hospital! The nice thing about it was I got over four miles in, and I was completely entertained by drunk men in a hospital. What more could a girl want?

Dr. Mulvey frequently gave me a hard time about walking because he said I exercised more than he did. I wanted him to see how dedicated I was to increasing my strength. I asked him to release me early from the hospital. He told me the following week might be rough because I would be neutropenic and was at risk for running a fever. I tried to negotiate, but he was noncommittal. I held up the sign Gary had given me that read, "Don't make me open up a can of pout." He just walked away. The victory was almost mine. He met his match in this Alaskan girl.

I was lying wide awake at three o'clock in the morning wondering if the poison running through my veins the past five days had killed all the blasts in my marrow. Did I pray enough? Did I do enough to stop the leukemia cells streaming through the body that had betrayed me? My biggest question was why someone so healthy could contract this disease. I ate right, I took vitamins, I exercised regularly. Why couldn't my body resist the medicine I had taken after the needle stick?

But it wasn't just me: Logan was nine, he was healthy, he exercised, he ate right, and he was so good. He was so loved. Every day on Facebook, I saw stories about little children who had cancer and were fighting to live. I wouldn't pretend to understand why it happened. I wouldn't pretend I accepted it. There must be a cure for all of us. I had many friends who were fighting for their lives. It shouldn't have been *any* of us; yet it was *many* of us. I felt thankful my mom was a breast cancer survivor. I was so happy that many had had victory over cancer.

I wanted God to heal me so I could stay on earth for years to come and be a testimony for him. But if he allowed me to die, I knew it was for His glory too. I would never renounce my God. There are reasons for everything. We may not understand, and we may not like the reasons, but I knew that living in heaven for all eternity was the greatest reward we could ever imagine.

Dr. Mulvey came in around six o'clock that evening. I whined about how bored I was. What I was doing was setting the tone for a release in a week or so. To my surprise, he told me I could leave in the morning! My labs were good, I had no fevers and no mouth sores, and I was walking over four miles most days. He made me promise to check my temperature four times a day and told me I had to go to the clinic in Post Falls every day. I eagerly agreed! He went to the nurses' station to start the process. A few minutes later, he came back and said, "Do you just want to go home tonight?" I jumped up and started packing the month's worth of belongings I had brought.

I looked over at Patrick and saw the apprehension on his face. Mom had left earlier that day to surprise Dad on his birthday. Patrick had to be responsible for me on his own. He was scared.

It was great to be out of the hospital. I was nervous, but we were only a mile and a half away. I slept intermittently that first night but much better than I had in the hospital. It was hard to accept I couldn't do a whole lot, but I promised to be a good patient at the Idaho house so I could stay out of prison. By the time we got to the clinic the next day, I was feeling pretty rotten. I knew it must be hard for Megan and Dr. Mulvey not to say, "I told you so." I was very nauseated, tired, and feeling all around yucky. As I sat there, I fought back tears of frustration. How could I go from feeling so good to feeling so sick?

The answer was in the lab results. My ANC had gone from about fourteen hundred to three hundred. I was neutropenic again. Megan reminded me that she'd told me before that the first week is the easiest. I had chosen not to believe that. I was determined to be different. I was determined to be the success story they would talk about for years. It reminded me of Logan being upset his ANC wasn't high enough to go to the mall. I finally understood, Logan.

Each day I had to report to the doctor's office. On February 6, I was granted a pardon at the eleventh hour. When I first woke up, I was doing great except for a bit of nausea. But while getting dressed, I found myself completely out of breath and dizzy. The house we were staying in had a nice-size closet, and I went in there to dress. I had barely gotten my clothes on when a rush of dizziness came over me, and the room seemed to spin. I lay down on the wooden floor thinking it was the most comfortable floor I had ever been on! I stayed there for a while thinking about germs getting into my respiratory system but didn't have the energy to move. Finally, I mustered the energy to go downstairs. I was looking for something when another wave of dizziness hit. It was time for my appointment, and I figured I would need some fluids.

Patrick pulled up to the door to drop me off. He was going to run across the street to the hospital to drop off a thank-you note I had written to the nurses on One North. He asked me if I needed an escort up. I scoffed at the suggestion as I apprehensively moved toward the door. I looked back to see if he had noticed my faltering steps, but thankfully he had gone. I needed to go to the infusion room on the second floor. There was no way I was taking the elevator, as that would mean accepting defeat. I climbed the stairs and headed toward the door. I couldn't breathe, and the room was spinning. I swear I saw stars.

I collapsed into a chair and said, "I need a bed." Charlotte brought a wheelchair over. "I will walk!" I said. Then I said, "Never mind; I need the help." I had succumbed to temporary defeat. I got in the bed, and they called Megan to come see me.

When she arrived, I told her I was just looking for attention—I liked people fawning all over me. She grilled me good. "How long have you felt like this? Do you hurt? Are you eating? Drinking? Fever? Chills?" I answered her honestly, yet as usual she looked at Patrick and asked, "Is she telling me everything?"

Geez. I might have downplayed a few symptoms, but I was honest when asked. She ordered orthostatics. That's when they measure your blood pressure and heart rate while lying down, sitting up, and standing. I failed. I received a liter of fluids and then did orthos again. Again, I failed. Both she and Dr. Mulvey had come in by this time and told me they were on the fence about readmitting me. They were concerned that I was possibly developing an infection, even though I didn't have a fever. They took blood for cultures.

Dr. Mulvey asked me if I just wanted to go back in since he could admit me then, rather than having me call the on-call doctor the next day. I politely declined his invitation. He told me if I had any symptoms at all, I was going in, and it was nonnegotiable. To his surprise, I meekly agreed. I had the same conversation with Megan. If I failed orthos for the third time, I was going to the big house. I narrowly passed, much to my relief.

This incident illustrates the power Leuk had to play with my mind. On the one hand, I'd thought I was doing everything right to help myself heal. But when I got weak and dizzy out of the blue, my determination faltered. Once, while in the clinic, I was washing my hands in the restroom. I looked in the mirror and started laughing. I finally got it! No matter how much I blamed myself for the needlestick and taking the medication, I had gotten leukemia through no fault of my own. I had blamed myself for months. If only…I laughed as I thought, "Only you, Marre, could have a son die of leukemia, get stuck with a needle, and get leukemia yourself."

It was just the luck of the draw. My destiny, my fate, whatever. I didn't mean for it to happen, I couldn't prove the needlestick made it happen, but by gosh I was going to stop blaming myself! I laughed not in amusement, but in freedom. Guilt had no power over me anymore! Or so I thought.

I'm a big believer in naturopathic remedies. I had always taken vitamins and used essential oils. When I finished the last two rounds of chemo, I returned to my natural regimen to repair the damage done by the chemo. I had been asking about continuing the usage, and Megan had agreed to do some research. She checked with the pharmacist and told me that some of the ingredients were known to counteract chemo. My revelation that I wasn't to blame for my leukemia came to a skidding halt as I sat there fearful that I had caused my relapse by taking the naturopathic remedies. Megan might have only known me for four months, but she could read me like a book. "You did not cause your relapse!" she exclaimed. "Stop blaming yourself!" The peaceful feeling went away as I again began to feel shame that I had caused my sickness.

My daughter Meghan, who also can read me quite well, called. I didn't tell her I felt guilty, but I told her what I had learned about the vitamins and oils. She said, "Stop feeling guilty, Mom! You didn't cause this, and you need to stop feeling guilty."

You see, my friends, guilt isn't from God. I had dropped the glowing presence of God and allowed Satan to fill my mind with doubt and shame. I refused to further allow him to have that power over me. But for the grace of God, there go I: "As God's fellow workers we urge you not to receive God's grace in vain. For he says, 'In the time of my favor I heard you, and in the day of salvation I helped you. I tell you, now is the time of God's favor, now is the day of salvation'" (2 Cor. 6:1–2).

Twenty-Nine

Next Phase: Managing out of the Hospital

Being out of the hospital was fantastic. I had my usual concerns—I had low blood counts and needed fluids, and central line number four was in danger—but overall, I was managing fine. The need to compete and strive for physical fitness overwhelmed me again. Casey and Kelsey arrived for a visit, and I wanted to celebrate. I declared I wanted to go hiking. Casey and Kelsey looked at me like I was nuts as I marched up the hill breathing heavily behind my mask.

"Are you sure you want to do this, Mom?" Casey asked. I muttered a reply and kept going. After a bit, I looked back and said, "What, you can't keep up with a sickie?" I saw the look of uncertainty pass between them, and I was determined to prove I could do it. I walked as long as I could, but the mask caused me to get overheated. I admitted I couldn't go any farther, and we turned around.

Dissatisfaction hit me because I hadn't made it all the way to the end of the trail. I had to pray, "Lord, take charge of my life and remind me to stop when I am trying to control my situation. Help me to see this as an opportunity for you to guide my journey. Take charge of my life and remind me to stop when I try taking control back. I can't do this without you, God."

Every part of my life was different. I even viewed the world differently after my treatment. Whereas I used to have little fear (except for mice and heights), I became afraid of new things because I felt so weak and vulnerable. When I saw children, I no longer gravitated toward them. Instead, I quickly moved out of their path. They were loaded with germs and might have had recent immunizations, which could be detrimental to me if I was near them.

I remembered one distinct moment when Logan was going through treatment. We had our neighbor's little baby, MacKenzie, over, and Logan was holding her. As his grandfather and I did, he always gravitated toward the babies. I don't remember how it came up, but I had learned MacKenzie had just had her shots. I quickly took her from him and told him unfortunately he couldn't hold her for several days. He was devastated. I had taken normalcy away from him. MacKenzie's mom, Lisa, made a quick phone call to the doctor and found out it was a dead virus, not a live one. It was with great relief that I placed the baby back in Logan's arms. Crisis was averted, and I was relieved to learn I hadn't placed him in harm's way.

Despite my concerns, I refused to stop living. I wouldn't be placed in a bubble. I knew I could use common sense and control what I could. For a person who didn't like limits, I adjusted fairly well. The Serenity Prayer came to my mind: "God, grant me the serenity to accept the things I cannot change, courage to change the things I can, and wisdom to know the difference."

Some days I wondered how I could possibly feel so good after everything I had been through. Casey and I reminisced about Logan's treatment. It was a normal day for him to vomit, but I had escaped the nausea for the most part. Did that mean the treatment for ALL is harsher than the treatment for AML, or did it mean the poison wasn't doing its job killing Leuk? Maybe what kept me from being so sick was that so many people were praying for me, but they had prayed for Logan too. Our son had endured so much with such grace and dignity. I knew Logan was cheering me on to finish the race.

Thirty

ISSUES AND PROBLEMS

You know how people joke about not jinxing things by bragging? I was impressed with myself because I had escaped feeling poorly for the most part. All good things came to an end, though. I started running a fever, and I had extreme body aches. I had been awake most of the night and didn't tell Patrick how sick I was. It was time to make that call to Dr. Mulvey. I wanted to be courteous, so I waited until 7:30 a.m. to call him.

"You know you need to come in," he responded. I think I shocked him when I said, "I know I am really sick, and I am okay with that." Unfortunately, there was no room at the inn. One North was full. He said he would call the ER and have them ready for me. To my dismay, it was a clown show there. The woman at the front desk had no idea who I was and why I was there, and she had no intention of rushing me back and giving me a private room. She didn't care that I was neutropenic and couldn't fight infection. To her I was a number. I wanted to weep as I sat in a wheelchair fighting to stay semi upright. Every part of my body hurt. I sent Dr.

Mulvey a text, and soon I was ushered back. I was thankful he had the power to make things happen.

Patrick and I were taken to a room in the emergency department, and we stayed in there for four miserable hours. The CNA wanted me to get into a hospital gown, but I adamantly refused because I was shivering so badly. I literally thought my body was going to fall apart bone by bone, muscle by muscle. Despite my pleas, they wouldn't even give me extra blankets because they were afraid my fever would go higher than the 103 it was. I felt as if I had arrived at the gates of hell. At last I was taken to a room on One North. I barely glanced around before I collapsed in the bed. I slept the whole day.

Despite my pain and sickness, it was time for the scheduled bone marrow aspiration. It was my fourth bone marrow biopsy in four months. I despised them, mostly because it seemed so unnatural to have someone drill in my hips. Thankfully, they didn't really hurt that much when Megan did them. Mostly they were just uncomfortable. I lost track of days while in the hospital. I know I was in there on Valentine's Day, and my mom made us a wonderful dinner with sugar-free apple pie for dessert. It was good to have Mom with me again. She and Patrick took turns staring at the four walls while I slept. My homesickness continued, and I broke down crying when talking to Granny. I missed my home, my friends, my animals, and my work.

My most recent PICC line had to be removed again. My central lines were not lasting long. I argued with the new patient escort when he tried to get me to lie down on a gurney. I was nothing if not stubborn and resistant to following rules. I insisted on walking in the procedure room again, much to the delight of the team who was putting in my fifth central line.

Waiting for the news about remission was difficult. I prayed, "Lord, I ask you to keep reminding me that *you* are in control of my life. When I have fear, give me courage. When I have doubt, give me belief. When I have weakness, give me strength. I know you will never leave me."

I got angry with myself when my mind raced at night because of worry. I wanted the peace of the Lord to calm my mind. It wasn't that I lacked faith; rather I wondered if God would choose to heal me. He gives and takes away. Thoughts raced through my mind. What was His desire for me? How could I serve Him best? Here on earth or in heaven? Why me and not Logan? Why do bad things happen to good people? They just do. I wanted to shout from the rooftops that God had healed me. I wanted to live the rest of my days declaring His glory. I declared that I would do that no matter the outcome.

I spent several more days exercising, attempting to sleep, praying that my counts would come up, and fighting the desperate feeling of imprisonment. I wish I could say I sat back and patiently waited, but that would not be truthful. I was blessed to have so many visitors break up the monotony of hospital living.

I entertained myself as best as I could. Our friend Rick bought me a great fur hat and fur slippers. I paraded myself around the unit and the halls like a model on the runway. I was certainly skinny enough to be a model! No matter how much I ate, I couldn't gain weight. I dreaded Megan coming in each day because I knew I was going to get "the lecture" about eating more.

I plotted daily about how to convince Dr. Mulvey to release me. It might have worked if Megan hadn't acted as a shield to my charm. She could deflect it like Superman deflects bullets. Gary tried to get me to see things from Dr. Mulvey's and Megan's points of view. He said, "I could take my BMW anywhere to get the oil changed, but I take it to the same place because they know my car and can foresee a problem and take care of it before it becomes worse."

Something finally clicked with me: I had great continuity of care. To interrupt that, for a short season in my life, might end up being detrimental to my health. I hurt because I wanted to go home so badly, but I knew my medical team had my best interest at heart.

I received another blow when a representative from Mayo Clinic called to inform me that no one matched me on the bone marrow registry and my brother's stem cells couldn't be used even as a half match. I felt rejected and alone. Why did both Logan and I have this issue? Were we that unique? Desperation and hopelessness were setting in.

After Logan died, I had organized several bone marrow drives. His friend Caitlin had registered on one of the first drives I coordinated. In just a few months, she was told she was a match for someone. I have always been thankful that because of Logan, someone else would live. I wanted someone who had registered in his memory to match me. It seemed that everything would come full circle if this happened. One of my nurses confided in me that she was a childhood survivor of both leukemia and lymphoma. She'd had a bone marrow transplant several years prior. That certainly encouraged me.

I was sinking back into depression. I needed to cheer myself up, so I had a Nerf-gun fight with one my nurses, Andrew. He wasn't my nurse that day, but he came in to visit me. He told me he had planned to come in earlier and jump on my bed to try and scare me, but my current nurse, Michele, had threatened his life if he woke me up. He wanted to pay me back for some of the tricks I had played on him. I would spend hours trying to come up with plans to torment my nurses. I had learned from the best. Logan was a tricky little thing and always plotting.

Despite the fun times, hospital life really was a drag. I was no longer allowed to make my own decisions, and I had no privacy. All modesty had disappeared out the window since I had become sick. One person after another would come in my room each day to listen to my lungs and my heart, check my pulses, and ask me if I had had a bowel movement. That question was usually asked in front of all my guests. I would often have a CNA on one side checking my vitals, while a nurse was on the other side messing with my IV. The CNAs would put the thermometer in my mouth while the blood-pressure cuff was on one arm and a finger on the other hand had the device to measure my pulse and oxygen. That left the CNA to hold the thermometer in my mouth. It made me feel like a newborn calf getting a bottle of milk.

I was chained to Tad like a dog is chained to a doghouse. I felt like a prisoner who was chained to a wall to prevent escape. Some days I felt as though I was literally going insane. I had to find humor in my situation, or I was going to go over the edge. I had no control over anything anymore. It was not a good feeling. I told myself, "Suck it up, Marre." Truthfully the walls were closing in on me. But the biggest battle was still ahead, so I needed to regroup and get my head on straight.

I had to be on guard against self-pity, and would often recite these lines for inspiration: "I wait patiently for the Lord; he turned to me and heard my cry. He lifted me out of the slimy pit, out of the mud and mire; he set my feet on a rock and gave me a firm place to stand. He put a new song in my mouth, a hymn of praise to our God. Many will see and fear and put their trust in the Lord" (Ps. 40:1–3).

The bottom line was that no matter how frustrated or disappointed I was, I couldn't change my circumstances. What I could do was change my attitude. I had to be thankful for what I had and remember to be grateful I was alive and able to share my life with family and friends. I was determined to have a grateful heart.

Despite my desire of a grateful heart, frustration set in yet again. My blood counts wouldn't cooperate at all. They would start to rise, then go back down, only to rise again and fall again. It was tough. I think God had a spectacular way of reminding me to be patient and trust in him. I had to remember to hold on to God and not try to focus on the future. I reminded myself that I must live for today and that it was okay to be hopeful, but it wasn't acceptable to worry. If we worry, we are saying we don't trust God enough. As Matthew 6:27 reminds us, "Who of you by worrying can add a single hour to his life?"

Dr. Reaves came in and encouraged me. He reminded me I'd had so much chemo that my body was fighting itself to make those healthy cells. None of my medical team members had given up on me, so why should I give up? I refused to live in the darkness. My nurses were quick to know when I was sinking into depression. Everyone wanted to see me beat Leuk. Logan never gave up, and neither would I. It was out of my control. The battle belonged to the Lord.

Thirty-One

FREEDOM!

Dr. Mulvey finally paroled me and started texting me at 6:45 a.m. the morning of my release to ask what medications needed to be refilled. What an amazing man and doctor. My counts weren't great, but my medical team felt that I would do okay at our Idaho house. When we pulled up to the house, Ringo saw me from the window and began crying like a baby. There is no feeling like the one you get when you realize your dog thinks you are the best thing since raw steak! He would hover as close as he could to me. I was limited in my activities, but much to his delight, I was permitted to take him for walks.

I kept visualizing and praying for my marrow to fill with healthy cells. When would it happen? I knew it was God's timing and not mine. So many thoughts filled my mind: Would I be in remission? Would a match be found? Would I get to go home? Would Olivienne remember me? Would my job be held for me? Those were the thoughts that kept me up night after night. Sometimes I was stubborn and held on to the worry. I turned into my granny, who always said she was up all night long worrying about someone in the family.

I didn't want to be a worrier! I wanted to be content with whatever God had in store for me, as Psalm 20:4–5 tells us to be: "May he give you the desire of your heart and make all your plans succeed. We will shout for joy when you are victorious and will lift up our banners in the name of our God. May the Lord grant all your requests."

I knew that God should be put first and that I should never desire anything more than Him. I knew I couldn't let my desire to go home be more important to me than building a closer relationship with Him. I asked God to fill my heart with peace and comfort as I eagerly awaited the decision about returning home.

I spent my birthday in the clinic getting fluids and platelets. I wanted to feel special that day, but not one single medical provider I saw acknowledged my birthday. I have always been a huge fan of birthdays. I like to make a big deal of them and sing happy birthday to the birthday guy or gal. Alas, there was no celebration for me at the clinic. But I did hear from many of my Alaskan friends and my family, which cheered me up.

Mom and I celebrated by taking a nice day drive to Kellogg, Idaho. We enjoyed the small town and walked around. That night there was a knock at the door of our house. We weren't expecting anyone, so I felt afraid. It was dark outside, and I was too weak to protect my mom. My first instinct was to reach for my gun, but I didn't have it. I knew I didn't have the strength to physically fight off an attacker. I warily opened the door, and four women I call my

"Cowgirl Pals" were standing there with a cake, birthday presents, and Minnie Mouse ears! I put on my wig so I could look decent for the pictures! Oh, the joy in my heart from feeling so loved overwhelmed me. I was truly blessed by so many people. Despite the distance from home, I was never alone. There was always someone around who wanted to show that he or she cared about me.

The care our home community continued to show us was incredible. Multiple bone marrow drives were being planned in my honor. Channel 11 news (Anchorage) aired an interview they had done with Patrick, Meghan, and Angelia Wilson. They showed pictures of Logan and told a bit of his story. My incredible husband shared his emotions in such a touching way. I just couldn't imagine how hard this was on him. First Logan and then me. I knew it was harder on my family than it was on me. I felt so thankful to have such a wonderful community surrounding our family. We knew God sent many earthly angels to support us, and we gratefully accepted their help.

Things were moving along. I finally got an appointment with Mayo Clinic. I was told to report to the ninth floor of the Charlton Building to pick up my itinerary. They made it sound as if I were going to a conference rather than participating in a bundle of medical tests. I was told a bone marrow aspiration would be done that day and was asked, "With anesthesia or without?" Anesthesia? Dang, I was tempted! I'd had five with no anesthesia, and it seemed wimpy to start using anesthesia after that many. It's like giving birth without an epidural for five children and then having one for the sixth. When I told Mom and Megan, they told me I was crazy for not taking advantage of it. I am not sure why I felt I had to prove I could handle pain.

We didn't have much time to prepare for the trip. Megan suggested we buy a one-way ticket since my return to Idaho would be uncertain. I stared out the window and gave thanks for the beautiful, sunny day we were having. I imagined the sun kissing my skin as I took a long walk with Ringo. I got up in anticipation, and my heart started beating rapidly, and I had trouble catching my breath. I knew instantly what the issue was; I was extremely dehydrated again. I just couldn't drink enough to keep my body hydrated. It was supposed to be my day off from clinic. I wanted to go for that walk, but I decided to be responsible and called the clinic to schedule a time to go in.

The next few days were busy as Mom and I packed up the Idaho house. We would not be going back to it. Mom would fly home with Ringo and I would join them after my visit to Mayo Clinic.

Thirty-Two

MOVING FORWARD

R eality hit me when we arrived in Rochester. I wanted so badly to avoid this step, but I didn't have a choice if I wanted a chance to live. It was great to be reunited with Patrick. He flew in from Alaska, and we met in the Minneapolis airport. He was very positive and encouraging. I made him promise that he would take me home for a visit whether I was in remission or not. It was hard not knowing what was ahead.

My emotions went up and down like a roller coaster. Sometimes I felt positive, and other times fear would take hold. I felt sadness wash over me when I said good-bye to my mom and Ringo. They had become two constants in my life and I was afraid to continue this journey without them. I knew I would see my mom again, but I wasn't sure I would live to return to Alaska where Ringo was going to be. Mom was amazing—always taking care of things and supporting us in so many ways. I had never felt as if I had taken my health for granted before, but I soon realized I hadn't appreciated how well my body worked before Leuk came in.

I was an emotional wreck waiting for my first appointment. It turned out that my blood sugar had dropped to forty-four, which explained part of my sadness. They sent in the "crash team" to take care of me. I felt it was a little much; I just needed some sugar! Because my blood tests had to be done fasting, I wasn't allowed to eat until they took the required seventeen tubes of blood from me. I never could figure out why they didn't have diabetics do their blood tests first thing in the morning.

The next day we spent over ten hours at the clinic. I had an electrocardiogram, chest x-ray, sinus x-ray, renal testing, a meeting with the bone marrow coordinator and doctor, IV fluids, and more blood tests. I got the news that there were still no blast cells found in my marrow, but we yet didn't know if I was in remission. I was told I could go back to Alaska for a week or two, which made my heart soar. I needed the break to mentally prepare for what was to come.

We had been apprehensive about leaving our small clinic in Idaho. Mayo Clinic was massive, but we quickly began to get used to the big facility. We found the people we encountered to be very compassionate, and we were thankful for that. I felt so weak and exhausted, and it was difficult for me to walk. Dr. Hogan suspected that my bone structure might have been affected by the twenty-pound weight loss. My thighs were so skinny that I could put both hands easily around them. The mirror mocked me by showing me how sick I had become.

I dreaded my upcoming spinal tap. They had to make sure my spinal fluid was free from leukemia before the transplant was done. Logan had had many of them, but up until my appointment with Mayo, I hadn't had to have one. I was thankful they permitted Patrick to be with me, as he was an amazing support. He never complained about all the sitting and waiting, and he always found something encouraging about the news we were given. He asked what would happen if I didn't have a transplant. Dr. Hogan was blunt and said I would have very little chance of survival without one. Leuk was very aggressive and he wanted to kill me. We had to arm ourselves with medical technology, strong medications, and radiation to fight back. I told myself that Leuk was not a worthy opponent. He was strong, but we would defeat him.

The next day was an eleven-hour day. When I reported to the check-in desk, I was told to go to room three. I sat in a cold room and was ignored. I was feeling nauseous and had a slight headache from the lumbar puncture the previous day. My life was not my own anymore. I felt disgusted when I looked in the mirror and saw a shell of the woman I used to be. I felt so vulnerable and fragile. As I walked to Station 74, I decided that no matter what I looked like, or how I felt, I would believe I was healed. I would no longer walk in fear. I would believe and trust God no matter what my body tried to tell me.

I kept thinking about my job and how much I missed it. I fought back the panic at the thought of losing it. Not only did I miss the work and my coworkers, but the thought of losing our medical insurance was also extremely concerning. Patrick had not signed up for insurance with his employer and couldn't do so until the following year. We only had insurance through my employer. I worried that we were going to lose everything if I wasn't covered. I kept telling myself to trust God and know that He would provide for all our needs.

After keeping a mundane schedule for so long, the next day we decided to be spontaneous and carefree. For a moment, we could imagine we were just a couple people going on a day trip. To me it was like finding the pot of gold at the end of a rainbow, because we were going to be reunited with our friends Tim, Diane, and Jennifer in Altoona, Iowa. Back in 1998, while at the Ronald McDonald House in Seattle, we had met Tim, Diane, and their children, Jennifer and David. I was instantly drawn to this neat family. They were warm, kind, friendly, and just plain nice.

When I gazed into David's eyes, I saw nothing but goodness just flow out of him. The feeling was almost tangible. His *soul* was filled with goodness. He reminded me so much of Logan. I had watched how he and Logan treated the younger kids. They were both so kind and were loved by everyone there. David had Ewing's sarcoma, which is a bone cancer. He had received treatment at Children's Hospital, but they were told there was nothing else the doctors could do for him, so they had returned to their home in Altoona, Iowa.

I will never forget the day David died. I grieved for him, and my heart hurt so badly for his family. The young, beautiful boy with his kind, transparent soul was gone. I hesitated to tell Logan. I wanted to protect him from the pain of losing his friend. But I decided he deserved to know. I called other members of Ronald McDonald House out to the garden, and we held our own memorial service for sweet David. Four months later, Logan joined his friend David. Both boys loved to fish, and I think about them fishing and hanging out in heaven just being boys and having fun. It was good for us to be reunited with David's family. No one can understand the pain of losing a child except another parent who has lost one.

The reprieve was too short. We had to drive back to Mayo for more testing. The first meeting the following day was with the radiologist who would determine the rate of the total body radiation I would have before transplant. Radiation was what I had been dreading the most. I remembered Logan's experience with pre-transplant radiation. He had gotten very ill with a migraine and vomiting. It was important that they used the highest dose of radiation my body could tolerate without being permanently damaged. All cells in my bone marrow would die before transplant. I was told that I would have radiation two times a day for three days, just before transplant. They measured my bones so that they could "custom fit" the radiation doses.

Although they never found a match for me on the national registry, they did find two cord bloods that would work. History was repeating itself, as that was what Logan received too. The good thing about using cord blood is there is less risk of graft versus host disease. GVHD occurs when the new stem cells attack the body, telling it that it's a foreign entity and that they are in control. GVHD can cause mouth sores that go all the way into the organs of the body, skin rashes, eye issues, and so on. These can be temporary or permanent. Some people are disabled for life after having GVHD. The bad thing about getting cord blood is that it takes longer for engraftment, so my immune system would be suppressed even longer.

While in Rochester, we searched for a place to live. We knew we were going to be there for at least four months and needed a house close to Mayo Clinic. Adult bone marrow transitional housing was available, but we didn't want to stay there for a couple of reasons. First, it reminded us too much of Ronald McDonald

House. RMH was an amazing place to be when Logan was sick, but the memories would keep flooding back if we stayed at this house, and I didn't think any of us could face the emotions. Second, only one caregiver was allowed, and we knew that we might have several visitors at the same time. We found a lovely home just seven blocks from the clinic and became friends with the owner. We were relieved our housing was secured.

Thirty-Three

HOMEWARD BOUND

The highlight was when I got to return to Alaska for a bit. I was home where hopes and dreams were both realized and denied. Casey and Kelsey picked me up, and it felt so good to be back with them. I took notice of every familiar thing: the roads, the houses, and the beautiful mountains that stood tall and proud. When we pulled up to our house, I felt the satisfaction of knowing I was home again. So far, I had survived! I was back in the home where we had raised our three children—the place where laughter intertwined with sorrow on occasion. My house wasn't just a building; it was a home. A home where I could be safe. I was content.

Both dogs were so excited to see us, and of course both had to sleep with us. I had almost forgotten what it was like to have to mold my body in a twisted position so my babies could sleep comfortably. Despite the yoga positions they forced me in, I slept well, as my mind could shut off and relax. In the morning, I sat there thanking God for His faithfulness. Without Him, I wouldn't have had this psychological break before transplant.

I had to laugh when my brother started texting me about staying away from sick people. He even posted on Facebook that no one should be around me if exposed to a sickness and that everyone must wash their hands before touching me. Mom wrote a note and taped it to my door stating the same things. She even bought hand sanitizer for people to use and wipes for the doorknobs. It felt so nice to be loved and cared for. They were 100 percent right; I simply couldn't be put in danger from an illness. I couldn't imagine being home and stuck in a hospital instead of sleeping in my own bed. That would stink!

I spent my first day with my daughter, granddaughter, and Granny. I had so much fun, but I was exhausted! Who knew a nineteen-month-old could wear me out so much? Granny spent the day with me because she worried I would overdo it. It was good to be home. Part of me couldn't even imagine that it was possible again. I visited with many friends and family members and even got to escape to my favorite place, our Kasilof cabin. I felt as if I had woken up from a horrible nightmare. All the months away faded in my memory since I had returned home. When the panic settled in, I rebuked it away and told myself I was living in the present, not the past, and not the future.

On April Fool's Day, I got the call I had been waiting for regarding my transplant date. The news certainly took me by surprise. Transplant was delayed for six weeks. I was thrilled I could stay in Alaska until the beginning of May, but I was also worried because I hadn't had chemo since the beginning of February. I was worried that the cancer would come back. The good news was I could work and attend Kelsey's nursing pinning ceremony.

I continued writing in my blog which helped me sort through my feelings and process what was happening. *This is an excerpt of what I wrote on February 17, 2015:*

I'm struggling, not in my faith, but just in torment of not knowing if I get to stay here and serve God, or if I get to serve Him in heaven. Whatever happens, I will serve my God. I'm not going to pretend I understand why this is happening or why it's His will. But I know He loves me. I know I have a home either with my family or in heaven with the Lord and Logan. Lord, I pray your favor upon me. I pray you bless me. I pray you give me remission and let me finish this process and survive. I want to be an example for you forever. You are a wonderful counselor, the way, the truth, and the life. You reign over all, and you are an amazing God.

During the time home, I struggled with low counts and low energy. I tried to do all I had done before Leuk invaded my body, but it was difficult. One morning I picked up some medicine to help with my mouth sores. Going to get the medicine was mentally hard for me. I didn't like going out in public because I was embarrassed about wearing a mask and a hat with no hair underneath. I went to Walgreens and got in line behind a woman. I had prayed no one would say anything to me. She turned around and said, "I was where you were eight years ago." She went on to say that she was impressed that I was going into the community because she knew it could be embarrassing with all the stares. It was as though she was reading my mind. She told me I was beautiful. Her comments brought tears to my eyes. She said she would be praying for me. What an awesome thing she did for me. I wondered if I would be so bold when Leuk was dead and I was cured.

Things were going well until Dr. Hogan called and told me I had to go back to Mayo Clinic for bone marrow biopsy number seven. He said I needed to be doing chemo soon since there was a delay in the transplant. He was concerned because my counts still hadn't recovered.

Would I ever be able to resume my normal life? I was lying in my bed trying to soak the memories in. The following week I would be so far away from my beloved Alaska. I dreaded leaving my family again. I was already homesick before I had even left. I was scared, but my family and friends shared with me that they were confident everything was going to be okay.

One of my friends wrote me the most touching letter, which included these words:

I really don't think you understand the profound effect you have had on so many people. Your courage, strength, and continued loyalty to all is very impressive and for me has impacted my life. Knowing how caring and giving a person you are and then to see you going through your current trial and tribulation and you continue being a hard charger focusing on the mission. Still giving, still caring, still Kelly!

Then he handed me something that touched me to the depth of my core: his Medal of Valor for his military service. This gift was from a true American hero, and he felt I was worthy to carry it on my journey. I was overwhelmed and honored to take care of it. I looked forward to the day I could hand it back because I was well.

I was invited to a prayer group by my dear friend, Lynda. Lynda is a beautiful woman who has always been on fire for God. She was a great support to us when Logan was sick. I will never forget her compassion. It was extra special because it hadn't been that long since her husband, Jerry, had died from cancer. I was always amazed that she had the strength to reach out to us. I was astounded at how many people came up to me at the prayer meeting to tell me they were praying for me.

God is so great. So many people in my journey to destroy Leuk were filled with His presence. He sent His workers to encourage me: "Truly I tell you, if you have faith as small as a mustard seed, you can say to this mountain, 'Move from here to there,' and it will move. Nothing will be impossible for you" (Matt. 17:20).

In my mind I screamed, "Leuk, get away from me! You have no power over me. My God is bigger than you."

On April 13, I spent my day cuddling Ollie while trying not to think about leaving the following day. The next day, Mom went with me on the flight to Minneapolis, and we had a fantastic flight attendant named Donna who said she would be praying for me. I found it amazing how God orchestrated meetings between people.

Thirty-Four

My Third Visit to Mayo Clinic

I tried not to dwell on the fact that just a day earlier, I had been in my house with my family close by. First up was the blood draw, then bone marrow biopsy number seven. I gave in and agreed to have it under sedation. Sedation wasn't offered in Idaho so I had gotten used to doing them awake. I decided I didn't have to prove I was tough. I knew I was and decided to go for comfort this time.

Of course, I had multiple tests and doctor visits to attend to, but my mother and I took a break and went on a great road trip to Lake City, Minnesota. What a gorgeous day it was. It was in the mid-seventies. We found a Friends of the Library book sale and loaded up on used books to keep us occupied while we were in Minnesota. We sat down by the marina and read and then took a nice walk around the marina. It sure was good to have a day off from the clinic. I felt great and was confident that I would hear the words "you are in remission."

It was strange to think how much my doctor controlled my life. He would know the secrets of my body before I did. He would know if the last chemo in February had worked to put me in remission. He would make the decision of what to do depending on whether Leuk was dormant or not. I had to stifle my strong personality and allow him to take charge. He was the expert on fixing people.

I had intimate knowledge of two people with leukemia: Logan and me. I had witnessed the experiences of dozens of others but had walked the path only twice. My doctor has treated hundreds, if not thousands, of people in my situation and could use those experiences to make the appropriate decisions for me so I could live without leukemia. I had to trust him. Thankfully there is a greater physician than my doctor, and I trusted Him completely. God always knows the secrets inside of me.

Although the test results didn't come back right away, Dr. Hogan seemed confident I was still free from leukemia. He told me I could go home to Alaska for two more weeks, and I was overjoyed. We celebrated this great news in New Ulm with our friends Lisa, Jerry, and MacKenzie Wanberg. We had a nice lunch together, and then we all walked around the charming town. We stopped in a Catholic church and admired the beauty. We went to Flaundrau State Park, and Lisa and I walked four miles on a trail through the woods. We spent our time catching up and sharing our appreciation for God's grace with one another. I was thrilled that my Fitbit showed I had put in six miles total that day.

Mom and I stopped for dinner on the way back. We were surprised when the waitress told us our meal had been paid for by a stranger. Mom and I were just about in tears. Even the waitress was about to cry. We were so touched. People were good. We packed up and flew back to Alaska.

Thirty-Five

HOME AGAIN!

On April 20, I got the news we had all been eagerly awaiting. I was officially deemed in remission. For two weeks, I could lead a normal life at home with my family and friends.

The following day I got up for work. Anticipation of the day ahead got my heart pumping fast. I was going to be productive for a change! No waiting around between labs, doctor visits, testing, or pharmacy. I was going to give something, rather than take. I felt joyful to be a contributing member of society.

For a brief moment, I allowed myself to feel the normalcy of it all. Then I looked at the dogs and imagined how they were going to feel when I left them again. My heart sank. Was it ever going to be real again? Was I really going to be all better and return to the life I had before? I happened to like my life. I knew there was no way of knowing if the treatment ahead would debilitate me or set me free. I tried to ignore these thoughts and regain my happiness and confidence.

Killing Leuk

On the way to work, I was listening to a Christian station, and the DJ said, "Sometimes you may think you can't go on because you have been sick so long. But if your heart is still beating, you continue on fighting and trusting Jesus." That resonated well with me. The verse in one of my favorite songs—written by Matt Redman—goes like this: "When the darkness closes in, still I will say, 'Blessed be the name of the Lord.'" Yep, it was time to buck up and soldier on. God is good, and work was going well.

I was shocked at how tired I was after working. I refused to use my treatment as an excuse. I attempted to continue exercising, but each night I was ready for bed before eight o'clock. I loved being at work but felt a twinge of regret every time I saw my fellow officers put on their vests and holster their guns. I missed going out to do field visits. I kept reminding myself that I was fortunate just to be home and able to process paperwork.

My heart sank as I looked at the schedule for my pretransplant appointments. Reality sat in. On May 12, I would begin full-body radiation twice a day, which would go on up to May 14. I was going to be in the hospital on Mother's Day. In 1998, Logan was also in the hospital for chemo on Mother's Day. He made me a gift in the hospital activity room. I remember being grateful that I was with him that day. I also remember being sad that I wasn't with Casey and Meghan. I wasn't going to be with my children, my mom, or my grandma this next Mother's Day. But with the sadness came relief—relief that the next step was approaching, because the sooner we started, the sooner we would be done. Leuk was going to fry—sizzle to his death.

While driving home that afternoon, I was thanking God for all the blessings He had given to us. I had done so well during all three rounds of chemo. Except for my line infection and blood clot, I had never had to return to the hospital because I was sick. I had tolerated the chemo and could continue my exercise regime. We were blessed with a place to live in Idaho and had a fantastic medical team taking care of me. My family and friends visited often. I had my dog with me! We had received financial gifts and loads of other gifts, including an endless supply of hats. We were prayed for and loved on. There had been several bone marrow drives held in my honor (and Logan's memory) so others could be helped with a match. We had been surrounded by our community, family, and friends. Our friends Carol and Mike organized a prime rib benefit dinner for me. They had done the same thing for Logan. *Many* of our friends helped with the event. We felt loved. So what if I was sick; a lot of people were. I wasn't going to sit around feeling sorry for myself. God was healing me, and I would forever give Him the glory for all the good and be thankful that He was there during the bad times. He was always faithful, and I would honor Him by being grateful and appreciative of what I had.

Patrick and I decided we needed a reprieve from it all. We decided to escape to the cabin and were delighted to take Ollie with us. When we got there, I strapped all twenty-seven pounds of her on my back and went for a walk. It felt good to push my limits, and I knew my heart and lungs needed to be strengthened before the next round of chemo. We were only able to stay one day, and the sadness washed over me when we left. I wasn't going to return to my happy place for months.

• • •

A friend asked me if I ever yelled and cussed at God because I had leukemia. I can honestly say no, I didn't. I wasn't mad at God at all. I didn't like having leukemia, but it wasn't God's fault. I knew He would hold me close throughout the entire journey of killing Leuk. I knew God was using my experience to make a difference in someone else's life. There was a purpose to my journey even if I didn't understand it. I knew that good was coming out of my situation. I only had to see how many people had registered for the bone marrow drive to be sure of that.

I had another friend whom I'd met only a few years ago. When she found out about Logan's death, she came to me with tears streaming down her face and said, "F—— God! How can you believe in God if He killed your son?" Oh, did I ever pray before I responded. Many people have asked me how I kept my faith all these years when God could have saved Logan.

My faith is so strong I never felt anything but trust in Him. I don't understand it, and I don't like it. I do not understand why, but who am I to question God? When I was diagnosed with leukemia, this same friend came to me and said, "Aren't you cursing God and saying 'F—— you, God'? Why you? You are one of the nicest people I know. Why did God do this to you?" I responded, "God didn't do this to me. But He will be with me every step of the way, and I trust Him."

• • •

I t was time to say good-bye to everyone. My coworkers had a "Good Luck / Au Revoir" party to celebrate the little French baby cells I would be receiving. (I had learned that the umbilical cords had been donated by a couple in France.) I attended church one last time and went for the last hike I would go on for a while. I kept telling the voice inside of me that it wasn't the "last" ever, just for a bit. My friend Kathy Conn gave me a beautiful cream-colored prayer shawl with branches of colorful leaves on it. She brought it back from Israel. Kathy is a breast cancer survivor. When Logan was sick, she and her husband Allen flew to Seattle to spend a week with us. She told me she put my name in the Wall at Jerusalem on two occasions. This was an amazing blessing, as Israel is the Holy Land and a favored nation of God. What an exciting gift for me to receive.

Patrick left Alaska before me because he had to fly to Spokane to pick up our car and drive it to Rochester. I had to fly by myself and be brave for what was to come.

Thirty-Six

TRANSPLANT TIME

I had many more appointments to prepare for transplant. During one of them, I was given a piece of paper informing me that my transplant would cost $400,000. I was thankful I had insurance and hurt for those who didn't. I couldn't imagine how it would feel to know that if you couldn't pay for treatment, you might simply be left to die.

Patrick and I had a disturbing, yet necessary, conversation with my doctor. He wanted to know if I wanted "full code" if there was a chance I could survive. He explained that if I agreed, they would just make me comfortable and let me die if I had something like a brain bleed and wasn't going to be "me" ever again. That's what I agreed to. Save me if you can guarantee I will be okay. Let me go if I won't be "me" again. I had no desire to be a burden on my family. Living in a vegetative state was not an option for me. I would rather be free in heaven.

Gary joined us for the big event. I was glad he was there to amuse Patrick, because the radiation about did me in. I had remembered how sick Logan was before his transplant, and I soon knew how bad it could be. It was certainly the worst of all the pre-transplant procedures. I had been dreading the urinary catheter, but that wasn't as bad as the radiation. I thought of my friend Mari who had a catheter for years. The three days I had one were nothing compared to what she went through. It is so easy to focus on our own problems, but when we turn our eyes on Jesus, the negative turns to positive. My eye was on the beholder, and I knew He watched over me. I had to remind myself to be grateful for all the medical interventions and not be angry for my body being subjected to heinous methods of treatment.

In the middle of the storm, I thanked Jesus. The battle caused my faith to grow immensely. I knew I had to stop trying to be in control and allow God to take over. He was a much better captain. I was ready for my French babies. I had a lot to live for, and I was eager to begin my new life.

God often uses the weak to accomplish His purpose. I knew this, so on the day of my transplant, I told myself, "I will not panic. God is with me. I trust Him." And I thought about these comforting words: "Those who know your name will trust in you; for you, Lord, have never forsaken those who seek you" (Ps. 9:10).

By two o'clock in the afternoon, my transplant was complete. Those baby cells fused through my body. There was nothing spectacular about the process; the cells were hooked up to my Hickman line and flowed through my body as many prayed over the procedure. I was thankful for the two sets of parents from France who had donated their babies' umbilical cords so I might have a chance to live. Patrick and I celebrated by dancing to "our song"—"Sea of Love"—in the hospital. We celebrated the gift of new life.

I got released to our rental house shortly after the transplant. I had to use a dry-erase board to keep track of all my medication. Some had to be taken on an empty stomach and at least an hour from the other medications. Some had to be taken two hours after consumption of dairy products, and others with food. It was a challenge to remember it all. I knew that was nothing compared to what was going to take place. I was warned I would soon be sicker than ever. I had to go to Station 94 every morning, and if I needed transfusions, I also had to go back in the afternoon.

I spent my days being pumped full of fluids and antinausea meds. I had reached "nater" with my white blood count. I was zeroed out: no immune system. The day came when I asked for a wheelchair. That was a difficult moment for me when I had to admit I couldn't walk to the elevator. I was continuing to lose weight, and my blood pressure was extremely low. I was nauseated and miserable. I was counting down the days to one hundred. I hoped to be released for home one hundred days after the transplant.

As I grew wearier, I turned to my Bible. These verses resonated with my soul: "Why are you in despair oh my soul? And why have you become disturbed within me? Hope in God, for I shall again praise him for the help of his presence" (Ps. 42:5). "Therefore, I will look to the Lord: I will wait for the God of my salvation; my God will hear me" (Mic. 7:7).

I prayed this prayer: "Thank you, Lord for the continued heal-ing in me. I trust you. I have hope. I believe. Please be with all my friends who are sick. I pray for complete healing for them." I knew I was going to be completely healed despite the rough process.

May 23 was a terrible night for me. I cried out to God and told Him I could really use a break. Everything hurt. My right shoul-der muscle and right side of my neck were excruciatingly painful. I tried ice, I tried heat, I had Patrick rub it—all to no avail. My throat hurt even worse. I consumed maybe five hundred calories that day. I understood how Job felt when he had so many calami-ties. I cried out to God and asked Him to help me: "Answer me when I cry to you, Oh my righteous God. Give me relief from my distress; be merciful to me and hear my prayer" (Ps. 4:1).

The nurse practitioner took one look at me the next morning and suggested admittance to the hospital. I, of course, said no. Then she wanted to look at my throat, and I started vomiting. I was embarrassed because our friend Tony was with us and witnessed that brutal moment. I agreed to be admitted. I spiked a high fever and had body aches and chills. I was told I might be in the hospital for two weeks. The doctor said I was going to get worse before I got better. I dreaded knowing that "rock bottom" was coming.

I soon found out how awful it was. My nights felt like I had been transported to the very gates of hell. The fevers continued, I continued vomiting, and I developed a strange rash from head to toe. My stomach and feet were very swollen. I had terrible back and shoulder pain and my jaw was hurting. My blood sugars kept bottoming out, but I couldn't keep anything down. I was having extreme pain in my sinuses, so a CT scan was done. The worst moment was when I was told that they had to stick a camera up my nose to see if I had a fungal infection. I feared the worst then, since Logan had died of a fungal infection after undergoing the very same procedure I'd just had. Thankfully the test was negative.

In less than a week, I had gained fifteen pounds from all the fluids. I was bloated and covered with red dots. There was nothing attractive about me, but beauty no longer mattered. Survival was my goal. I was in excruciating pain, but thrilled to hear that on day fourteen I had begun to engraft.

The nausea was probably the worst of it. I had mild GVHD in my gut, which explained the intractable nausea. Graft versus host disease is a terrible condition that many have after transplant. I describe it as the new cells coming in and saying to my body, "You don't belong here! This is *my* home now, and you have to leave." A great battle takes place, and the battle wounds can be fierce and deadly. Cord-blood transplants are less likely to cause GVHD than adult-cell transplants. As bad as it was, I was thankful it wasn't worse.

I was released on June 4 after eleven days in the hospital. When my nurse practitioner told me how well I was doing, I promptly burst into tears. All I could think about was how well Logan had appeared to be doing too. He had fought like a champ, and I knew I didn't deserve to live any more than he did. Yet I was fighting so hard to remain with my family and friends. Why should I be spared? But I wanted to be. In times of trouble, I have always gone to my Bible. This verse seemed fitting for the battle I was fighting, ""Praise be the Lord, my Rock, who trains my hands for war, my fingers for battle. He is my loving God and my fortress, my stronghold and my deliverer, my shield, in whom I take refuge, who subdues peoples under me" (Ps. 144:1–2).

I had so many visitors and rotating caregivers. I loved every one of them. My friends and family loved on me and tried to cheer me up. The day Meghan arrived with Ollie was icing on the cake. Ollie ran in saying, "Grammie's here, Grammie's here." She sure could pick my spirits up quickly.

There is no hopeless situation, I realized. Our hope is our anchor: "We wait in hope for the Lord; he is our help and our shield. In him our hearts rejoice for we trust in his holy name. May your unfailing love rest upon us, O Lord, even as we put our hope in you" (Ps. 33:20–22). My hope continued to be in him.

As I struggled with the sickness, I prayed this prayer: "Lord, you know my limitations. You know how I feel. You know I'm not afraid to die, yet you know how badly I want to live and serve you here. My life isn't going how I would have chosen it to go, but you are with me. I will accept your calling for my life."

I began dreaming about getting a fungal infection as Logan had. I couldn't control my dreams, but I wished I could. I wished I would just dream about Logan being healthy. I wanted him to guide me through the process of recovery. I was fighting to live and was thinking about addicts who didn't value life enough to fight for survival and freedom from addiction. My heart was burdened for the hurting. I had so much time on my hands, and I started thinking about how I could help others when I was better. I realized that some of the hardest things I had been dreading were successfully completed. Radiation, having a catheter, not brushing my teeth for a month, and so forth—I had completed it all and was doing okay. The things I cared about—the hair, eyelashes, and eyebrows—were gone. I didn't care how I looked anymore. I proudly displayed my bald head. I had earned it! I knew I was going to be okay.

When Logan was sick, he asked me to find a verse in the Bible to comfort him. I needed comforting too and often read this passage to help me through the process. This is what I chose for him, but it also became a comforting verse for me: 2 Corinthians 1:3–7:

> Praise be to the father, our Lord Jesus Christ, the father of compassion and the God of all comfort who comforts us in all our troubles, so that we can comfort those in any trouble with the comfort we ourselves have received from God. For just as the sufferings of Christ flow over in our lives, so also through Christ our comfort overflows. If we are distressed it is for your comfort and salvation; if we are comforted it is for your comfort, which produces in you patient endurance as the same sufferings we suffer. And our hope for you is firm because we know just as you share in our sufferings, so also you share in our comfort.

Thirty-Seven

KEEP ON GOING

I wish I could say the remainder of my one hundred days' post-transplant was uneventful and a breeze, but it wasn't. For those of you who may be reading this because you want to know what is ahead for you or your loved one, I *wish* I could tell you it was easier. But I *can* tell you I survived it, and the pain and discomfort of what I went through has faded from memories.

I continued to have problems with my central lines, fevers, and viruses. I was put in the hospital a couple of more times, and I still struggled with weight gain. When I was diagnosed, I weighed 137 pounds. At my lowest, I dropped down to 101. I was so skinny that my skin literally hung off my body. I looked like I was ninety years old. I had elephant skin. It was disgusting, and I hated looking in the mirror. I had always taken care of my body, and my body had failed me. I really struggled with self-image, and I tried not to. I tried to focus on my spiritual life, not my physical life.

Killing Leuk

I was getting cranky about halfway through those hundred days. I wanted to do what I wanted to do, not what my doctors and caregivers thought I should do. I was sick of being poked, prodded, and lectured. I was done with it all. I just wanted to go home. I wanted to live again. I kept telling myself that my new lifestyle wasn't going to last forever. I felt ashamed for complaining when so many people were much worse off than I was.

I tried to just focus on how much love had been shown to me. God blessed me in so many ways. He protected me, healed me, comforted me, and certainly loved me. He provided me with genuine people who remained in contact with me and supported my family and me through the whole process. No, I had no right to whine or complain. The road traveled was long and difficult, but I believed Leuk was dead and not lying dormant, ready to pounce again…

I knew from the beginning that my attitude would be crucial to survival. When I was told I had a rare form of leukemia, I was calm and ready to slay the intruder. I knew if I fell apart, my family would too. I refused to put them through anything harder than it already was. Attitude was a choice. I could continue to strive for good health because I had the strength of the almighty one. I kept singing this verse: "My eye is on the sparrow, and I know he watches me."

I prayed this prayer shortly before I was released to go home:

I trust you, Lord. Your will be done, and you will see me through this. Give me the courage to resume the activities I desire to do in our community. Give me strength to get through each day. Please bless all my sick friends who are also fighting life-threatening diseases and may also be anxious and scared. Help me be a blessing to others. Please bless my family, who loves me and supports me, and wants me to live here on earth for years to come. Heaven will be incredible, but I believe you have more work for me here right now. Help me to trust and resist the fears. Guide my local doctor to recognize anything of concern. I love you, Lord, and I thank you.

I also recited Romans 15:13: "May the God of hope fill you with all joy and peace as you trust in him, so that you may overflow with hope by the power of the Holy Spirit." I had joy, and I had hope, I believed. I accepted my journey, and I trusted my God.

I was so weary. Two days from going home to Alaska, I was admitted back to the hospital for uncontrolled nausea. I used my amazing manipulative skills and was released in time to catch my plane. The nausea was manageable and I was going home.

Thirty-Eight

HOMEWARD BOUND AGAIN

We flew from Minneapolis to Seattle. As we landed in Seattle, my heart began to ache. To this day, I still struggle with many emotions when I think about Seattle. I remembered how we left Logan there after his spirit left us. We flew home to Alaska, and our son's body was still in Seattle. My heart hurt because I was alive and our son wasn't. I grieved that he didn't make it a hundred days posttransplant and I did. I grieved because I loved him and knew he deserved to live so much more than I did. Yet I knew I had to fight to live because God had a purpose for me. I knew Logan understood that.

We were greeted enthusiastically at the airport by my parents; my niece Michelle and her husband, Jimmy; and Casey, Meghan, Ollie, and Delanie. They held up welcome-home signs. I couldn't believe how surreal it was to walk off that plane knowing I was home. We had done it! We'd killed Leuk and I'd survived. I just wanted to go home and acclimate again.

I spent the next day unpacking all my suitcases and boxes. Ollie got really upset when I picked up an empty suitcase. When I asked her what was wrong, she said, "Grammie can't lift that!" I said, "It's okay, honey; it's empty and not heavy." She said, "It's not heavy? Okay." She loved me so much, and at two years old, she understood that Grammie was sick and a little fragile. Knowing how much she loved me motivated me to continue fighting to survive. I wanted to show her that Grammie could be strong and normal like her other grandmas.

I went back to work on September 2, 2015—less than four months' posttransplant. I agreed to follow the doctor's orders and only work part time to start, but I had already let Dr. Hogan know my desire was to return full time as soon as possible. I worked that first morning and then drove myself to Anchorage for my doctor appointment. I stopped by to see my Anchorage coworkers and then went to the store. By the time I got to the oncologist's office, I was extremely nauseated. I had to get IV fluids and antinausea medication. Dr. Spencer's jaw dropped open when I told her I was already back to work. Everyone seemed astonished but me.

I struggled with the lectures of the many people who loved me. Everyone had an opinion about what was best for me. I appreciated the advice and the compassion, but I'd had enough of being told what to do for all those months of treatment. I was ready to do what I wanted to do. I just wanted to be normal again. I didn't even *know* what my new normal was. I just wanted to pretend nothing had ever happened to me, but when I doled out my daily pills, I realized that was an impossible task. I wasn't normal. I had handicaps and limitations. I wasn't the same, and I was frustrated. I discussed my feelings with a friend who'd had a liver transplant. We shared our frustrations at not having the energy to do what we were used to doing. We both wondered if we should push ourselves to get stronger or if we should slow down. Neither of us knew what was right.

My Anchorage oncologist, Dr. Spencer, said I couldn't go to church because too many sick people attended. I couldn't be around wood stoves, and I couldn't be around anyone who had recently had a live immunization or had recently been sick. I was still wearing the Vog mask that Mayo Clinic had recommended. It's a mask made from cloth and I could wear it for thirty days before replacing it. There are many different designs to choose from, which made it a little fun. One of my coworkers named it Bane. I ended up having to wear a mask for about thirteen months' posttransplant. I couldn't even go outside without it on. I hated that mask, but I dutifully wore it because I knew it would protect me against fungal infections and other illnesses. I felt like such a freak when I went to the store and people stared at me. I was continually being humbled by my appearance. My clothes hung on me, and I looked like a child dressed up in adult clothes. There was nothing attractive about me. My hair started growing back slowly, and to my dismay, it was gray instead of brown! I couldn't even dye it because it was too fragile. That just added insult to injury there. I wasn't even allowed to wear makeup because it could cause GVHD to flare up on my face. If you ever think you need a touch of humility, try cancer treatment. It humbles you.

On September 14, 2015, I made a note in my blog:

Happy four-month posttransplant to me! Four months ago, I got umbilical cord stem cells from two unrelated donors from France. In four months, I have made great progress and really feel well. I walk between 1.5_3.5 miles per day, do eighty squats, forty-five wall push-ups, and some other miscellaneous exercises each day. I am working four hours per day and trying to organize my house a little bit each day. I make dinner most nights and pack Patrick a lunch. All the things I used to do. Does it ever feel good! I say this not to brag, but to share how good God is and how He has helped me overcome all the bad. I feel very positive, optimistic, and hopeful that I will survive. I believe Leuk is dead forever thanks to our faith and trust and God's mercy. There's not a moment that goes by that I'm not thanking God for every single living thing.

How little did I know that things were going to get bad again in just a few months.

Thirty-Nine

New Symptoms

On September 24, I made my first trip back to Mayo Clinic. Of course, I insisted on going by myself. I am nothing if not independent and stubborn. I went out to dinner that first night and was called "Sir" by two people. The very short hair and no makeup made me look like a man. I was embarrassed and humiliated. I was lonely and sad and wished I had someone with me. My appointments went fine, and I returned home two days later.

I was exhausted from the trip, and a new symptom had started on the airplane: my legs felt weak and numb. As the weeks went on, the symptoms continued, and it felt as if I had electric shocks going up and down my legs. I began to feel very frustrated with myself and struggled with being positive about the strides I had made. I was still struggling with nausea, reduced stamina, and various aches and pains. My weight was still fluctuating, and I was being lectured about the need to consume more calories. I finally figured out that I had developed an allergy to nuts. Peanut butter and nuts had always been a favorite for me, but I noticed that every time I ate anything with nuts in it, I would vomit two hours later. After "experimenting" with this a few times, I concluded I could never eat nuts again. I kept telling myself that it was more important that I was alive, so not eating nuts wasn't that big of a deal. But to this day, I am still lamenting my nut-less diet.

The issue with my legs greatly concerned my doctors. I had to have a spinal tap and an MRI in Anchorage. The results were inconclusive. No one had an explanation for what was going on. They were concerned that I had relapsed, but thankfully that was not the case. I continued doing the best I could at home and at work. I went to Anchorage for a meeting and ended up curled up on my boss's bench in his office because of extreme nausea. It wasn't my finest hour. He called Patrick to come and get me. I felt like I was doing the walk of shame when I left. I was humiliated and felt like I couldn't pull my own weight. I knew I was a burden on my coworkers, and I struggled with my inadequacies. I wanted to be back at work in full capacity. I struggled with guilt for being sick. There was a war going on in my head, and the devil taunted me that I was inadequate.

On October 24, 2015, I reflected on the anniversary of Logan's death. It had been a Saturday night, and he had struggled all day. I had suspected it was going to be the day he left us. Not a moment goes by that we don't still feel the pain of losing our firstborn child. A year before, I was in the hospital alone after receiving a similar diagnosis. I remembered a part of me welcoming death because I could be with Logan again. I had shared my feelings with one of my nurses, who had the compassion to sit and cry with me. But a year later, I was still here and knew that I had to honor Logan by continuing to get better. We didn't want to dwell on our grief, so Patrick and I took Ollie for a drive to Talkeetna. We knew how much Logan would have loved to have been an uncle.

Six days later, we were overjoyed to meet our newest granddaughter, Meghan's second child. Ailynn Claire was born at home with more hair than I had. She was beautiful and simply perfect. We were overjoyed to have another granddaughter to love and spoil. We discovered that the pain of losing Logan wasn't ever going to go away, but having two grandchildren to love did help us heal. I felt blessed to still be alive to hold our second granddaughter.

Because I seemed to continuously catch illnesses, Dr. Spencer called and told me she didn't want me to have any contact with our granddaughters. I had been compliant with all the conditions my doctors had put on me, but this was one request I wasn't going to honor. What was the point of living if I was ostracized from the precious girls who I had fought to live for? I had to trust that God would protect me and keep me safe.

I celebrated my six-month posttransplant anniversary and wrote this in my blog:

I have been in a mighty battle. Swords have been raised against me, I have been poisoned, and radiation has killed my old marrow. Yet here I stand, six months later, shouting in victory. I am alive! It hasn't been easy, and I have been discouraged many times, but I serve a faithful God and He sends His messengers to pick me back up and send me back into that battle, a little stronger than the day before.

I continued to have some issues with my lungs, and in December, my doctors again told me they suspected I had a fungal infection. There was nothing like hearing the words that they thought I had the same kind of fungal infection Logan had died from. Patrick and I headed back to Mayo for more testing. I had several days of testing done, which was unpleasant and stressful. I had tubes stuck down my throat on two separate days, I had my nerves shocked and needles placed in my legs, I developed a fever and chills after the bronchoscopy, and I was poked and prodded endlessly. I was very relieved when we got the results that I did not have a fungal infection. We were thankful and happy, yet my heart hurt because in just a few months, I had lost several friends to cancer. I felt guilty for surviving, and I struggled with the joy of my success when they had tried just as hard as I had to survive.

Forty

Full-Time Work Approved

On January 5, 2016, Dr. Hogan reluctantly agreed to allow me to return to full-time work. I still wasn't released for field duty, but I could work full time again. One more step toward normalcy!

Even though I went back to working full time, I was concerned about my energy level. I was still struggling with insomnia and didn't have much energy, but I was determined to show everyone that I was a survivor. My weight was up to 110 pounds, and things were going well. I was still exercising and was feeling well overall.

More requests came in asking me to speak with people who had been diagnosed with cancer. Of course, I readily agreed to be a support to others. From the very beginning, I said I would use my experiences and journey to comfort others. I modeled my attitude after my favorite verses from 2 Corinthians 1:1–6:

Praise be to the God and Father of our Lord Jesus Christ, the Father of compassion and the God of all comfort, who comforts us in all our troubles, so that we can comfort those in any trouble with the comfort we ourselves have received from God. For just as the sufferings of Christ flow over into our lives, so also through Christ our comfort overflows. If we are distressed, it is for your comfort and salvation; if we are comforted it is for your comfort, which produces in you patient endurance in the same sufferings we suffer. And our hope for you is firm, because we know that just as you share in our sufferings, you also share in our comfort.

Those words comforted both Logan and me. We were not alone in our sufferings because we knew Jesus suffered with us. But He was also there to comfort us, and it was my pleasure to help others along similar journeys. My biggest desire was to be a real and true example of someone who walked the walk, not just talked the talk.

Working full time exhausted me. I tried to retain high spirits, but I started planning my funeral. I decided that I wanted my service done my way, so I picked out which songs I wanted sung, who I wanted to officiate the service, and what I wanted done with my body. I told myself that I was just being a control freak like usual—that it wasn't because I thought I was going to die anytime soon. I told a few people what I was doing and asked them to stand up at my funeral and make fun of me for continuing to try and control things from the grave.

My February checkup with Dr. Hogan went very well, and he released me for full duty. I was ecstatic and couldn't wait to tell my boss. Imagine my disbelief when he refused to allow me to go back in the field. Josh was an excellent boss, but he cared more about me than he did about my job. He didn't think it was safe for me or my partner and wouldn't let me go in the field yet. I was so disappointed, but I understood where he was coming from. I decided that I would transfer units so I would no longer be a hindrance to my coworkers. We only had two officers in the house-arrest unit, and I was a detriment to the office due to my inability to perform all my duties. Arrangements were made for me to transfer to Palmer Probation, since there were more officers who could cover my field visits until everyone felt it would be safer for me and my fellow officers.

Forty-One

Very Bad News

Things were going well until I got sick again. Patrick and Ailynn had colds, and although we were careful, I was still exposed. I developed a sore throat and terrible wheezing in my lungs. I had no energy and thought I was just being lazy. *In my blog, I described how I felt like this:*

> I did hard time in prison (hospital) for a VERY serious offense. I got put on discretionary parole for good behavior, and I took positive strides to better my health. I was doing well on discretionary parole and got this misdemeanor conviction. This misdemeanor conviction is an irritant and worrisome. Will it mess up all the good things I have accomplished on parole? The "misdemeanor" (cough and body aches) doesn't seem like a big deal, but combined with my very serious felony conviction, I am concerned. But I didn't just find God in prison. I have known Him my whole life and will continue to trust Him.

My forty-ninth birthday was on March 10, 2016, and my birthday present was admittance to the hospital. It was officially my worst birthday ever. My misdemeanor turned into three felonies. I had three respiratory illnesses; RSV (Respiratory syncytial virus), coronavirus, and pneumonia. RSV is usually seen in babies, but my immune system was like that of a newborn baby and susceptible to infections. I was very sick. I continued to be stubborn, however. That morning I still tried to get up and go to work, but I could barely raise my head up. I told Patrick I needed to go to the doctor. My doctor's office said they couldn't get me in until the afternoon. I knew it was bad and needed to be admitted to the hospital. I insisted Patrick drive me in right away. The ride to Anchorage was horrible because I felt so sick and uncomfortable. When we got to the parking garage, I started dry heaving. I wasn't supposed to be out in the air without Bane. I had no choice but to rip the mask off. I could barely walk into the building. I sat down in the middle of the elevator.

I dimly remember others walking in and Patrick apologizing for me. Part of me wanted to tell him he shouldn't have to apologize because I was very sick. The other part of me didn't even care. I remembered the time I was six years old and had had encephalitis. My mom had stopped to clean up my vomit in the hallway, and all I wanted was to lie down.

Zack, my PA at Alaska Oncology, took one look at me and said, "Do I need to admit you?" I immediately answered, "Yes." Then he looked at my SAT rate and said, "There's no doubt about it, you are going to the big house."

The doctors at Alaska Regional Hospital contacted Mayo Clinic, and a treatment plan was agreed on. Two days later, I was moved to the intensive care unit. My lungs had been badly attacked. I reacted poorly to one of the IV drugs and almost got intubated.

I had to wear a BiPAP mask that delivered pressurized air to my airway. It kept my throat muscles from collapsing. It was similar to the one Logan had worn at the end. It was a very uncomfortable and claustrophobic. It dried out my mouth so badly I couldn't even move my tongue. They wouldn't allow me anything to drink or eat. I had severe anxiety issues. Even with the oxygen, my SAT rate was only 95 percent. I was scared and honestly felt like I was going to die. I almost felt glad that I was finally experiencing what Logan must have felt. I had some regrets at leaving my family but thought, "At least they won't have to worry about me anymore." I was asleep more than I was awake.

I had a dream about God. I dreamed there were many of us walking—apparently on another plane. It wasn't earth; it wasn't heaven. Suddenly we all stopped and gazed in wonder at the sight before us. God was revealing His kingdom one snapshot at a time. It was overwhelmingly beautiful. I was left knowing there was more, but that was all I was going to see at that moment. Many tried to take pictures with cell phones, but the phones wouldn't open to the cameras. We knew God would not allow us to share this with others who weren't there. We waited in a seemingly prearranged spot. God Himself was coming down to tell us what He needed us to do for Him! Unfortunately, I woke up before I saw Him. How special I felt to be one of the chosen ones.

Forty-Two

Finally Released

I was released after thirteen nights in the hospital. I went home and had to be on an oxygen tank for the next few weeks. I was not happy about being hooked up to the tank, but I was so thankful that I had survived my latest ordeal and could sleep in my bed again. What I didn't foresee was that the illness would take away my job, and I would once again be wondering what the purpose for my life was. I wasn't even allowed to hold my grandchildren because I might catch another illness from them, or spread my germs to them. I couldn't even be in the same room with them.

I was distressed and broke down in tears. I had fought so hard. I had beaten Leuk. I'd had a successful transplant. I was back at work and getting ready to soon go back to the field. And I got a stupid cold? It had ruined my career! A stupid cold! A stupid cold that turned into RSV, coronavirus, and pneumonia. I was angry. I loved my job. God had other plans for me, and I had to accept it, but I deeply grieved my losses.

Ollie came to visit. She knew the rule about staying in the doorway, but she was not happy about it. She said, "Why can't I come in your room? I want to hold you, Grammie!" She would inch a little farther in the room and say, "Grammie, say Ollie get out of here!"

I tried explaining to her that the doctor said I could get babies sick. She then made up symptoms to show she was already sick so she could be with me. It made me happy and sad at the same time. The next day I had a complete emotional breakdown, and Patrick had to stay home from work to take care of me. I was supposed to be the strong one, the self-sufficient one, the independent one, yet I cried like a baby as he helplessly stood by not knowing what was going on. Why couldn't being alive be enough? I wasn't allowed to work, clean my house, or hold my babies. I wondered what good I was to anyone. I was terribly lonely.

Once again, I turned to prayer: "Oh Lord, forgive my doubts and fears. Help me to appreciate all the blessings. Let me see the good in all things. Direct my path how you want my life to be. Use me to be a blessing to others. I trust you have my future mapped out. It may not be what I had planned for myself, but your ways are best."

As my faithful husband continually told me, "This is a journey, and we will love every moment because we are together."

I didn't like "me" anymore. I felt like I was losing my mind. The hunter became the prey, the helpful became the helpless, the independent person became dependent, the confident became unconfident, and the happy me became miserable. It was like having a good angel on one shoulder and a bad angel on the other. One told me I was a child of God and still had many positive attributes, and the other told me I was worthless and unlovable. I wondered why I couldn't just be happy being alive.

My inability to just be grateful that I was alive was especially puzzling in light of what had happened to my very good friend Mari. Mari was a strong and vibrant woman who instilled fear in all those around her. She was powerful, smart, intelligent, and independent. Then Mari was diagnosed with multiple sclerosis, and within a couple of years, she was unable to walk or care for herself. This beautiful and vibrant woman was reduced to a bedridden person who was dependent on everyone to meet her basic needs. Mari quickly became bitter and angry. My children and I had visited her often, and we would take her to church with us. We tried to give her what she craved most: companionship. My heart hurt for her. I didn't see Mari much the last couple of months of her life. She had moved back to Anchorage, and I was busy. I didn't know she was dying. I will never forgive myself for not being there for her at the end. I should have been there.

Now, as I remembered Mari's last days, I knew I didn't want to be reduced to an angry and bitter person. Like Mari, I detested being dependent upon anyone. I wanted my husband to have a real wife who was independent and self-sufficient.

At a follow-up appointment, Dr. Spencer asked me how my spirit was. She knew. She ordered me (in the way only doctors can) to get Joel Osteen's book *I Am*. After listening to the first four chapters, I realized that God knew what was wrong, but He needed me to praise Him and claim healing upon my body and mind. I needed to affirm this with my words. I had to stop focusing on what I *couldn't* do and focus on what I *could* do. This was a season in my life, and it would end. Death would not defeat me, and my life wasn't destined to be one of constant medical issues. God was restoring me, and I believed that completely. I began claiming victory in Jesus.

I told myself, "I am healed. I am stronger. My family will serve God all the rest of our days. I am beautiful because I am a child of God, and He wonderfully and fearfully made me."

I am often asked, "Why is it always the good people who have such tragedy?" The Bible says, "It rains on the just and the unjust." In other words, both good and bad people are subjected to all sorts of things. It's what we do with our circumstances that defines us. Let's say we are given bad news or a bad medical report. What do we do with that? We should look to our God and pray for strength. It is true God will not give us more than we can handle. We are strong and mighty warriors in Christ. We should not sit around and feel sorry for ourselves. We should pick ourselves up off the floor, dust ourselves off, and go back in the ring. We are believers, and we are fighters. We are in the ring, and we will be the winners. When that bell rings, we will raise our hands up and give thanks to God for guiding us through the fight, the battle, and the worst thing we could ever imagine happening to us.

I finally realized that no matter what, God had known this was going to happen to me. He knew I was going to get leukemia sixteen years after Logan died. I can't even say I was shocked, because He prepared me two months prior to the diagnosis, just as He prepared me a few days before Logan was diagnosed. I don't want to sound like I'm some special person—more in tune with God than most—but I'm telling you, He talks to me, and I know ahead of time when something bad is going to happen. My spirit is connected to *Him*. I'm not sure if that's bad or good…Just kidding! I know it's good, but sometimes having a little bit of time when I feel at peace wouldn't be so bad! But I feel good knowing He prepares me.

It doesn't matter what we are going through—whether it's grief, addiction, an undiagnosed illness, an immune disorder, migraines, financial stress, worries about children, or anything else. Our job is to proclaim victory over the illness/problem and *believe* God will take care of it. Our job is to keep our faith and never give up the fight. Get back in the ring. The battle is not over. Remember Philippians 3:14: "I press on toward the goal to win the prize for which God has called me heavenward in Christ Jesus." And remember Philippians 4:13: "I can do everything through him who gives me strength."

Forty-Three

Finally, the day had come. I celebrated the anniversary of my first year posttransplant. I had made it a year! I was thrilled to be alive and relatively healthy.

Being the optimistic person I usually am, I hoped that when I visited Mayo Clinic for my one-year checkup, my doctors would change their minds about allowing me to work. After I'd gotten so ill with a cold a few months prior, they had forbidden me to work outside the home. But now, I secretly hoped Dr. Hogan would release me for work after all and that somehow I could retain my position as a probation officer.

I had multiple days of testing before I saw my doctor. Before my appointment, Mom and I flew to Indiana to visit our friends and family. We flew separately from Indianapolis to Minneapolis. Mom's flight was delayed so I was on my own that first day. I inadvertently consumed some nuts. I foolishly thought they were broken-up toffee pieces on my sugar-free candy. By the end of the day, I was curled up on a seat in the waiting room and trying not to vomit on the bench. Thankfully, I made it into the restroom on time. After my appointment, I got into my car and had to stop several times to vomit and I was embarrassed about it. Patrick later told me, "No one knows you there, so don't worry about it." Famous last words, as my nurse told me the next day that she'd seen "some lady throwing up at the stoplight." My face was red as I told her that lady was me.

My days were again filled with CT scans, chest x-rays, pulmonary function tests, multiple physician visits, blood tests, immunizations, and a bone marrow biopsy. There was no end to the torture. The bone marrow biopsy was either my tenth or eleventh—I'd lost count of the drilling that took place in my hips. My feet were so swollen that they looked like they belonged on a three-hundred-pound woman. I had multiple x-rays of my feet.

I was still convinced Dr. Hogan would release me for work after all, but he shot that hope down quickly. He said he would never forgive himself if I were injured on the job and he had released me. His words stung like a bee, and I had to take several deep breaths to compose myself. I was crushed. Wonder Woman had been defeated after all.

All the way back to Alaska, I conversed with myself and attempted to put a positive spin on my circumstances. I tried to be optimistic about the harsh reality of my circumstances. After all, I was alive, I could be flexible with my schedule, and I could volunteer, babysit our granddaughters, go to the cabin, visit with friends and family, and just enjoy life. I was determined that I would not lie down and wallow in the pity of self-despair even though I was disappointed with the curve ball life had thrown at me. I reminded myself that there are many who are much worse off than I was.

This was the prayer I prayed on my return home:

Lord, today I come to you to repent. I have focused so much energy these past nineteen months trying to get better so I could go back to work. You know how much I loved my job. My desire to return to it inspired me to exercise regularly and gain strength. I gave it my all. I trusted you for complete healing. Yet here I am with new symptoms that are concerning. I am told certain parts of my body have been damaged. No one can tell me if the damage is temporary or permanent. I cried out to you to fix me. But two weeks before my Mayo appointment, my symptoms increased rather than improved. Sometimes I must accept help to get out of a chair. My pride and independence are fading. Maybe that's your plan. I thought I was still dependent on you, but maybe my narrow focus made me think more about what I wanted than what you wanted for me.

I will not grow bitter for what I have lost. To the end of my days, I will cry out to you in gratitude. For you have given me the greatest gift of all, salvation. Salvation outweighs how many miles I can hike and how well I can shoot a gun. My physical abilities do not define me. My innate spiritual thoughts and eagerness to follow you do. Help me become who *you* desire me to be. Please show me and direct me on this new path. Help me not to be selfish, but to share my soul with others who need you. Please let me honor you however you see fit. I love you, Jesus, and I thank you for your love. Help me share my story to bless others. Thank you, Jesus. And please give Logan a hug from his momma and tell him he gives me courage every day.

Unfortunately, the bad news continued. The osteomyelitis issues I'd had in my jaw at the age of twelve were still bothering me. When the results from the recent CT scan came back, I was told my condition was severe, but there was nothing they could do for me because of my leukemia and recent stem-cell transplant. I was told that at some point I would need to consider pain management. I was forbidden to work in my yard or with flowers, and I couldn't dust or vacuum my house. I felt worthless.

I had to fly back to Mayo Clinic the following month because I was still having problems with my legs and couldn't get to see a rheumatologist in Alaska for at least six months. We had already spent a few thousand dollars on my Mayo trips and medical expenses just since the beginning of the year. I cried out to God and asked Him what His plans were for me. I knew God was in control and was holding me in His arms, but I admit I had daily emotional struggles. Every time I thought everything was going to be okay, a new symptom popped up. I was struggling with insomnia every night and was exhausted during the day. When I was in kindergarten, we had taken a nap every day. I reverted to kindergarten. Without a nap, I could not function.

Forty-Four

HOPE

That third trip to Mayo in 2016 brought me a little bit of welcome news. My doctor decided if I wore an industrial mask, he would give me permission to clean my house and work in the yard. People were astounded that doing menial work was so important to me, but they were people who had never been restricted from normal duties. No one could possibly understand how important executing menial tasks was to me. I was so thankful to have a little bit of normalcy in my life. Was I supposed to just "sit there and look pretty"? Not a chance!

In June, we celebrated Patrick's fiftieth birthday and our thirtieth anniversary. It was important to me to renew our wedding vows on the deck of our cabin. I had never been so thankful to be married to my husband. Patrick had taken his original wedding vows seriously; he had taken care of me in sickness and in health. He was in for the long haul, and I felt so thankful to be his wife of thirty years. We wrote our own vows this time around. When

Patrick read his vows, his words blew me away. I tear up every time I think about how much he loves me.

We held both parties at our favorite place—our Kasilof cabin. My mind always went to our "happy place" when I was stuck in the hospital. I wanted so badly to return there. It was the perfect spot to reflect on everything we had gone through in our three decades of marriage. We had experienced many rough times filled with disappointment, sorrow, and loss. But most of all, there had always been love. I have a sign in our kitchen that says, "Every love story is beautiful, but ours is my favorite." How true that is. I love my husband more every single day. I am grateful he stuck by me even on my ugly sick days. The love he showed me has solidified our relationship, and I know he will indeed love me eternally.

On June 24, we reflected on the special day of Logan's birth. He would have been twenty-nine in 2016, and our hearts were hurting. He was a sweet child—well mannered, easygoing, and very compassionate. He loved to bike; play soccer, basketball, and baseball; fish; do martial arts; hike; and spend time with his family. He enjoyed pretty much everything. He was a caring big brother and tried to look out for his younger siblings. He fought such a hard battle and would have won it if he hadn't gotten a fungal infection. I spent years blaming myself for not protecting him enough. I would still take his place if I could. I would take his place and let him live if only I had the power to do so. The world lost a beautiful boy, but heaven gained a beautiful soul.

I know that ultimately we will all die, and if we know Jesus, we will have the opportunity to live eternally in heaven. I know that

Logan must be having so much fun with his friends from RMH, Chris and David, plus the many others he knew and loved. Then of course there are his family members, including his cousin Matt, who recently joined him in heaven. I know Logan is having a good time, but it doesn't take away our pain and feeling of loss when his birthday is upon us. For years, it hurt so much that we struggled inwardly and silently grieved alone. In 2016, however, I convinced Patrick to take my dad, Meghan, and Kirk out halibut fishing to celebrate Logan's life. Logan loved to halibut fish, and Homer was his favorite place. Patrick expressed guilt about going on Logan's special day, but I told him there was no better way to honor our son than to catch a big halibut in his memory.

Forty-Five

GOD IS FAITHFUL

How do I share my faith with others? How do I convince people there is a God? How do I describe the miracles I have witnessed? How do I declare my healing has taken place because God is not finished with me yet? I have tried to be an example to everyone I encounter, but I have often failed. I have lived a long time and have had many experiences, which are not all good. Yet I still believe in God. God is the head and the center of everything. To my dying breath, I will proclaim His goodness and never deny Him.

I was given this life so that I may share my story and comfort with others while they are going through similar situations. That is what we are to do—share our experiences with others so that they may be comforted and know that there is a God who does care about them. It is our utmost duty to share with others. Some think I may be a little crazy for all the sharing I have done. But the support I have received from others has not just uplifted me. I also like to think that sharing my raw pain, discomfort, and turmoil, along with my praises, has uplifted others too.

Helping others gives us a sense of accomplishment and makes us feel good. Have you ever been going through something when someone mentioned that he or she had a similar experience? Did it make you feel good to know the other person made it through? That all was not lost and that you too can survive and thrive? I know that when Logan was sick, I yearned to hear about survivors of leukemia. It gave me hope. Although Logan didn't survive, I still needed that hope while we were battling the most terrible disease that was upon our child. Through our experience with Logan, we have been able to help others emotionally and financially and to educate the public. We have shared Logan's story, and many have registered to be bone marrow donors, and some have even saved the lives of others by becoming donors. We have raised thousands of dollars for cancer research and patient support. I say this not to boast but to urge you to make a difference in the life of another.

I have learned how important it is to focus on the ones who mean the most to us: our families. Our families need our attention. We tend to focus on many distracting things that really aren't important, and we don't spend the quality and insightful time we should with those we love the most. We spend a lot of time getting ready so we look perfect. We do our hair (I have hair now!) and our makeup, and we want to look just right because humans tend to want to focus on appearances. But we also need to focus on our hearts. I always told my children to pick a mate who was not only attractive on the outside but also on the inside. Thankfully, Casey and Meghan each found a person who is exactly that—beautiful on the inside as well as outside. But how much time do we spend working on our hearts and souls? Are we intentional with our thinking, or are we just focused on what others can see?

Outward beauty will fade, but beauty on the inside will always be noticeable. I think about this a lot, because I used to be one of those people who wanted to look good on the outside. I worked out, tried to stay in shape, spent way too much time on my hair, and so on. But did I spend enough time on my heart? I'm not saying outward appearances don't matter, because there's nothing wrong with looking good and taking care of your body. We need to take care of our bodies for health reasons, but we also need to take care of our hearts.

I want my family and friends to know how important they are to me. I want to speak kindly to them and build them up rather than put them down. We never know when we will be separated by death. I don't want to ever regret not saying "I love you" to those I love.

I continue to have days that are good and days that are bad. But I can find something good in *every* day, even if I must really look hard. I struggle with guilt for being alive when others aren't, and I struggle with limitations that have been put on me because of my immune system. The treatment has aged my body, and sometimes I feel like an elderly woman. At times, I need help getting to and from the floor, and frankly, I don't like that. I want to be "me" again. I want to be impulsive and carefree, but I can't. There may be a hidden germ out there ready to take my life away.

My fourth trip to Mayo in 2016 brought me more discouraging news; my doctor would still not release me for work. It's been a regular job just trying to keep my spirits and emotions in check. I love being able to volunteer, but even that must be carefully regulated so I am not exposed to an illness. Every day I tell myself to be the best person I can be to others and to myself. Yes, I must be kind to myself too. I must forgive myself for not measuring up to my own standards.

I'm always embarrassed when people ask me, "What do you do?" I try not to excuse my inability to work. It hurts when people say, "You don't look sick. I don't know why your doctor won't release you." Trust me; I *do* want to work. But God has a plan, and I must sit tight and wait until it becomes clear. I am ready to serve God and my community in any way "He" sees fit.

These past twenty years have been quite the journey, filled with both dizzying peaks and valleys as well as discouraging dead ends. On the one hand, I still have days when I am frustrated with my limitations and frequent illnesses. I used to have a fantastic immune system, but now I catch everything that comes around. I must fight off depression and work on having a positive attitude each day. But on the other hand, I have learned so much from experiencing the death of my child and surviving leukemia. I know what is most important in life. I know that life isn't easy and not always fair, but I've also learned that God never leaves our side.

I want to be a shining light in the darkness. God has been good and faithful, and I am blessed. Until the day He chooses to reunite me with Logan, I will love and appreciate everyone and everything around me. I am hopeful. I am strong. I am a warrior. I am an overcomer. God has healed me.